Advance Praise for
INFORMED, AWARE, EMPOWERED

Informed, Aware, Empowered is a must-have resource for anyone with a cervix and healthcare providers. This informative book walks you through female reproductive anatomy, and explains the significance of the often-ignored cervix in our menstrual and reproductive health. Denell shares invaluable and incredibly detailed information in this book about how cervical abnormalities develop and most importantly, what can be done to address those abnormalities through targeted lifestyle, energetic, food, herbal and supplement protocols. This is an easy-to-digest, comprehensive guide to cervical wellness and care that I recommend to all of my clients.

— Nicole Jardim, Certified Women's Health Coach and author of *Fix Your Period*

Informed, Aware, Empowered is what the women's health education industry has been waiting for, as proof of the healing power of holistic methods for HPV.

Nawrocki gently navigates the confusing diagnosis of HPV with both science and intuitive body wisdom, and empowers the reader by addressing taboo emotions of fear, shame and guilt around sexuality that can come up when receiving test results.

Her methods help the reader develop her inner medicine woman by accessing the voice of her body with self-inquiry, self-love rituals, and methods for creating healthy boundaries. In addition, it provides both education on the science of the immune system and options other than the HPV vaccine and invasive surgery to empower the reader to make informed decisions around her body's healing process, with options of nutritional, herbal and emotional healing practices.

— Allie McFee, Women's Health Educator at *Modern Goddess Lifestyle*

Praise for
DENELL NAWROCKI, M.A. AND
CERVICAL WELLNESS

Denell is a bright light of hope and resilience around this topic. She is one of the few people who served as a role model and gave me the faith that IT COULD BE DONE.
— Brie (reversed CIN 2/3 with high-risk HPV)

I couldn't have done this without you and I'm so endlessly grateful that I was led to you. Your work is so powerful. You helped me change my life. You bring so much light and happiness to so many women. You will always have a place in my heart.
— Sandra (reversed CIN 3)

THANK YOU DENELL…. Before finding you, I had no idea what the cervix was, let alone where it is located, and ALL THE REST!
— Leonora (Reversed CIN 1 and HPV 16)

You have helped me heal myself, and that is a gift that I will always carry and hold dear to me. You are a special soul and what you are doing is amazing. Words cannot express how much all of this means to me and how grateful I am.
— Aoife (reversed CIN 3 in 2 months)

Mother of Above:
I just want to thank you for supporting my daughter during her struggles with severe dysplasia. I am so grateful that she has healed and incredibly grateful that she found you. You are a true earth angel.

You're a modern-day hero.
— Audrey (partner of a client)

INFORMED

AWARE

EMPOWERED

INFORMED AWARE EMPOWERED

A Self-Guided Journey to Clear Paps

By Denell Nawrocki, MA

SMOKEBLOOD PUBLISHING
Casper, WY

SMOKEBLOOD

ISBN-13: 978-0-9600491-6-5

Library of Congress Control Number:
2019916133

Published by S M O K E B L O O D Publishing
Casper, WY | smokeblood.com
@_smokeblood

Cover design and layout by Colt McMurry
Cover design © Smokeblood, 2019
Edited by Marissa Waraksa

Book illustrations © Hillary Mendoza, 2019
wildmagik.com | @wild.magic

Printed in the United States of America

For my Grandmothers, Mother, Sister, future daughters,

and all people with a cervix.

CONTENTS

The land of healing lies within,
radiant with the happiness that is blindly sought
in a thousand outer directions.

— Paramahansa Yogananda

Author's Note

While I use the words *Woman, Women, She* and *Her* throughout this book, I want all readers to know that this information is pertinent and valuable for all those who have female reproductive anatomy, regardless of how they identify themselves. I support and advocate all those with cervixes to connect with and take care of this unique body part.

FOREWORD

IN 2015, a bodyworker had his finger on my cervix during a healing session. If you're not familiar with the idea of intimate bodywork, this could be quite confronting to read. But for me it's a very 'normal' experience. I was researching sexuality at the time and coaching clients into better sexual relationships with themselves. So this session was all in a day's work, you could say. What I didn't realize was that my cervix would become the focus of the session. I also didn't realize that this session would change the course of my life.

There, on a hot day in Bali, I discovered my cervix was numb. I devoted the next years of my life to trying to understand why.

Through my explorations and by listening to the testimony of thousands of women over the years, I believe the cervix is the next piece of our pelvic anatomy to play a huge part in female sexual awakening and empowerment. You see, the cervix is not just fundamental to birth, it is

1

also an independently orgasmic organ. Most people don't know this, including doctors. In fact, when I took a survey of people in the street in London, Berlin and New York, the cervix was mainly associated with birth, cancer and HPV. So from the outset, we're limited, simply because we don't have the information.

Then there are other factors. In order to access the cervical orgasm, we need to look at our personal conditioning as well as social structures that shame or disempower sexually alive and embodied women.

Not surprisingly, the orgasmic cervix has also been mostly ignored or marginalized by science, with outdated or inaccurate information still being taught in leading gynecological schools worldwide.

Many mainstream doctors and sex therapists will tell you *it's normal* for the cervix to be numb or to feel uncomfortable during stimulation. *Normal*, maybe. But not natural. This skewed perspective exists largely because of Alfred Kinsey's report from the 1950s, wherein he claimed his research participants were not experiencing sensation during stimulation, when in fact they were. Regardless, Kinsey's findings became the dogma that is still used today.

It wasn't until the groundbreaking work of Dr. Barry Komisaruk who, through his studies on women with spinal cord injuries, discovered that the cervix is capable of not only pleasure but also orgasm and that these orgasms have their own neural pathway via the vagus nerve.

In fact, the cervix is connected to three sets of paired nerves — more than any other part of our genital anatomy. The cervix is a very important organ, not only for birth, but also for its potential to generate some of the most transformative orgasms ever reported.

So, it made no sense to me that my cervix was numb. After that day in Bali, I had followed the instructions given to me by the bodyworker; but because of my numbness, I soon gave up. I had decided cervical stimulation was not my idea of pleasure. Nevertheless, driven by my own curiosity and renewed determination, I started an online group to provide mutual encouragement and support for anyone who might want to take on this practice alongside me, and thus continued to do the work.

What emerged from that group was eye-opening. I knew we were onto something. Women were releasing grief, rage, shame, memories, even past life experiences. They were also discovering a new part of themselves. A part that had been roughly treated, ignored, bumped, poked or pounded. They discovered that this part of themselves, hidden from the world, was also a gateway for personal development and pleasure. This is how Self:Cervix was born — a project providing online courses for cervical healing, activation and orgasm.

Through the sharing in the very first round of Self:Cervix, it became clear that the main causes of numbness and pain were premature penetration, birth trauma, disassociation and invasive medical procedures.

Women started coming out with all sorts of concerns and worries about how to deal with HPV (otherwise known as the 'common cold' of STIs) and cervical dysplasia, especially since the growing list of side effects from the Lletz/Leep made the procedure more than just 'routine' (These can include loss of libido and PTSD-like symptoms as well as numbness). And still, every week I'm approached by women who fear the consequences of the LlETZ/LEEP procedure. It seems they sense the trauma these procedures can cause, and they're determined to do whatever they can to avoid any kind of cutting or removal.

Advising on such things is a difficult position to be in. On one hand I want to tell people, 'don't do it unless you really need to' but at the same time, I understand what it feels like when your doctor tells you, 'if you don't, you could get cancer'. When I'd had cervical dysplasia, I remember I just wanted those abnormal cells gone. I didn't know I had any other options. It's one thing to talk about healing naturally, but it's another thing to figure out how.

That's when I came across Denell's much-needed work.

With little or no options for alternative approaches to healing cervical dysplasia and HPV, Denell became my go-to source. Denell's work provides a much-needed alternative so that women facing medical procedures can truly make an informed decision.

I'm so relieved that Denell and Cervical Wellness exists so that I can send women to her rather than offering only hope and a suggestion to reduce stress.

Perhaps through the application of her work, women will not have to go through countless colposcopies and multiple Lletz treatments. Denell is providing something of a savior to our cervixes and is advocating a different path which allows women to take control of their own healing and avoid mutilating their beautiful cervixes.

This makes her a disrupter of the system and a rebel for her cause. Much like me, the only way to create change is to question and challenge everything we take for granted. It is because of her bravery and determination to give the proverbial middle finger to the Lletz that Cervical Wellness now provides a haven for women seeking a healing solution.

And as you'll read in this book… this healing is not just topical — it's systemic. To heal such a core part of our being, we need to address all the many factors that contribute to disease in the body; in particular, our views about ourselves as women, sexual beings, healing grief and ancestral imprints. Just like the cervix, this work takes us deep inside.

I'm proud to be walking this path with Denell. We are like two beacons advocating for the cervix on different sides of the world, upholding different parts of the mystery. Because truthfully, the cervix is still a mystery. Because the science is limited, we only have experiences and testimony. It's a classic case of science vs spirit. Some things may never be proved. Sometimes it's just too hard.

So we embrace the feminine way. We feel it, experience it and know it for ourselves. Perhaps this is one of the most beautiful lessons of the cervix: The answers lie deep within. We are invited into our own authority. The cervix is a part of us that remains in the dark. So does its mystery, and maybe that's a beautiful thing.

Olivia Bryant
Self:Cervix

PREFACE | MY STORY

I choose to tell you my story of healing HPV and cervical dysplasia because it gives a greater context to this work. It provides an understanding as to the journey I traversed to help you see that your journey is perfect, and that you are exactly where you need to be right now.

Receiving the diagnosis of HPV and cervical dysplasia is scary, and it does take *time* to heal. Healing is a marathon, not a sprint, and in revealing my story, you will begin to understand why I choose to call it a marathon.

I invite you to receive my story, and to notice where it may mirror your own...

7

The first time I was told I'd tested positive for HPV, I was sitting in an exam chair at a Planned Parenthood in Sacramento, California. I was nineteen, and I remember feeling quite alone. There were one doctor and two nurses, each of them wearing yellow-colored scrubs. I remember hearing a baby crying on the other side of the door, and the smell of the chemicals they used to clean their floors.

I had never met the doctor who was seeing me, before that moment. When he told me I had HPV and cervical dysplasia, he didn't even look me in the eyes. He kept his head down, studying my chart (this was before computers were widely used in exam rooms) and said quite plainly,

"Your pap smear came back abnormal. You have HPV and cervical dysplasia. There's nothing to worry about. You're young. You'll naturally heal. Everyone has HPV at some point or another, and it should just go away on its own. You can go now."

Those words went in one ear and out the other.

What does that mean? I don't think that 'abnormal' is a very good word. I thought. *Oh well, I guess I've nothing to worry about since the doctor said so. I'll just go.*

And so I went, not giving my gynecological health another thought.

Little did I know that this dismissal of the state of my cervical health, along with the lack of information the doctor had provided to me, would set me off on a four-year journey of shame, fear, guilt, anger, regret and pain, followed by another three years of warrior-like determination to figure out cervical dysplasia.

Sometimes I wonder how different my twenties would have been, had that initial doctor explained to me what HPV was, what cervical dysplasia is, what they were actually checking when I went in for a pap, and ideally, a few pointers as to how I could support myself in healing. Instead, he sent me out the door with no more information than when I'd come in.

I left Planned Parenthood with the understanding that I didn't have to do anything differently, and so I went about my life. I continued my lifestyle as a fast-living college student, and continued to fill my time with beer-pong, late-night wild parties, academic stress, and processed foods.

After receiving the diagnosis of HPV and cervical dysplasia, Planned Parenthood advised me to routinely get pap smears. I needed to be seen every six months to have the dysplasia monitored. Over the next year and a half, I continued to receive the same diagnosis, and in that year and a half, not once did my doctors at Planned Parenthood tell me what anything I was experiencing meant or how I could help myself.

All I ever heard was, "You're young. You'll heal."

Once again, I didn't change anything. I still continued to live my life as a now twenty-something college student with the full knowledge that my cervix was unwell. I continued the party-girl lifestyle, having sex with multiple partners and not changing anything I was doing, because I trusted what my doctors had told me.

I graduated from the University of California at Davis with a degree in History, and moved back home at the age of twenty-one. No longer having access to the Planned Parenthood I had been going to, I searched out a health service provider with whom I could continue to have routine paps, and found a nurse practitioner with whom I felt really good.

Around this time, I entered into a new partnership. I told my partner I had HPV, and he wasn't too concerned with it. I chose to use a new birth control device called the Implanon, since I was in a new, monogamous relationship and didn't want to get pregnant. The Implanon is a hormonal device implanted in the inside of the upper arm that continuously releases the hormone progesterone and suppresses the pituitary gland, stopping the ovaries from releasing eggs. Little did I know that this choice would actually exacerbate the cervical dysplasia. None of my medical practitioners had told me this could or would happen.

By the time I found all this out, I'd had the diagnosis of HPV and cervical dysplasia for going on three years. In those three years, I had received four different colposcopies (biopsies of the cervix) and the dysplasia was actually getting worse. What started out as Cervical Intraepithelial Neoplasia (CIN) 1, had now progressed to CIN 2.

The new nurse practitioner I was now seeing was concerned with my prolonged diagnosis of HPV and progressive cervical dysplasia, and offered to perform the LEEP procedure or to provide me with the HPV vaccine. Neither of these options felt good to me. I wasn't willing to have surgery without anesthesia to remove a portion of my body (which may prevent me from being able to deliver a child naturally in the future due to scarification). It also didn't make sense to me to receive a vaccine for something I already had. I refused both options.

Another year goes by, and my diagnosis continued to progress. I endured another colposcopy biopsy and the results showed the cervical dysplasia worsening. I was now bordering on CIN 3. My healthcare providers were concerned with how quickly the cervical dysplasia was progressing, and advised me to come in to be examined every few months. They routinely told me that I was on the road to developing cancer, and continued to try to push me into the vaccine and the LEEP.

Still, I said "No" to both of those options.

Since I was refusing treatment, my nurse practitioner suggested I begin to take the supplements Folic Acid and Lysine. This was the only time any healthcare providers gave me any sort of lifestyle advice.

One thing I want to mention is how my doctors told me that, in order for me to heal, I needed to 'stop having so much sex'. I was also told that 'something was wrong with me because I wasn't healing' and as a twenty-three-year-old Woman, these were terrible words to receive from people I looked up to and respected. I became extremely depressed and anxious. I became fearful of my body, and began to harm myself by hitting my own body and uterus with my fists because I was so upset with what was happening. I felt deep shame about 'how much sex' I had had in the past, and developed a neurosis around sex and my sexuality.

I would find myself crying, puddled on the floor because I felt so ashamed that something was wrong with this portion of my body, and I had no idea what was happening. I didn't know what a cervix was. I didn't know what cervical dysplasia meant. The doctors would continue to say the big 'C' word — CANCER — to me, and that's all I could think about.

Around this time, I was sent away by my healthcare providers to another doctor because I was refusing the treatment options of the vaccine, the LEEP procedure, and cone biopsies. My regular practitioners told me that I needed to get another opinion because I wasn't 'listening' to them. I felt it was because they had become fed up with me. Since I didn't know what else I could do, I complied, and went to see an OBGYN in one of the larger teaching hospitals in my area.

I went alone to this teaching hospital, because I felt so embarrassed by what was happening. I didn't want to involve anyone else. In fact, I was alone throughout this entire story so far. Yes, my boyfriend knew what was happening, and yes, I had told my Mother and sister, but no one wanted to talk to me about it or asked how I was doing. This whole experience was very 'hush-hush'.

Now I'm at the hospital. I remember like it was yesterday. I was in a huge OBGYN teaching room at the largest hospital in my county, just me and the doctor. I could feel the enormity of the space around me as I laid there, exposed in the direct center of the room. All the student seats around me were empty, yet the space felt like it was filled with fear, shame, and regret. The air was cold, and my skin prickled in response. There was a sterile, stale smell to the air, and the room lacked ventilation. This was the least comfortable I'd ever felt in any gynecological exam.

In this exam I endured my **seventh** colposcopy biopsy with a doctor I'd never met before. As I lay in the chair, feeling the vast expanse of space around me, I began to wonder, *Am I a slut? Am I this person who just had too much sex? Is there something* **wrong** *with me? Why is this happening to me? What is happening?* All these questions and thoughts raced through my mind as she snipped off three more pieces of my cervix. I felt so, so ashamed.

After the examination and colposcopy, the doctor rolled around to the side of the exam table on her wheeling stool, and looked at me with worry in her eyes. She put her hands on my thigh when she came to my side. Her touch was gentle and warm, but it sent shivers down my spine.

What was she going to say?

She looked me directly in the eyes and said, "Denell, you refuse our treatment. The only options I can offer you are the HPV vaccine or surgeries, and you continue to refuse. **I'm sorry. There is nothing more we can do for you."** My heart sank.

That was the truth, right there. My doctors couldn't do anything for me. They couldn't help me heal. They didn't know how to support me in healing unless I had them remove portions of my cervix. I felt like I had been given a death sentence.

The words "I'm sorry", "Cancer", "hysterectomy" and "hopeless" floated around my mind as I quickly got dressed and rushed out of the room. Holding back tears, I left that hospital completely defeated. What was I going to do? If the doctors couldn't help me heal, then what? I'd hit gynecological rock bottom.

I erupted into tears as soon as I got home. I remember the shuddering and shaking of my body as I realized that these authority figures whom I'd looked up to and put my faith in for four years were literally leaving me out to dry. I collapsed into a puddle on the shower floor and prayed for help. I prayed that, at my young age of twenty-three, I would heal and still be able to have children, that my reproductive system would be healthy and well, and that I wouldn't have to worry anymore.

While lying on that shower floor, a light suddenly appeared in my heart — a glimmer of hope that I'd yet to have felt when it came to my HPV and cervical dysplasia situation. Something shifted within me with this spark of light. With the appearance of this light, I heard my body's voice for the first time. My body told me, "We are going to figure this out. Something is wrong, clearly, but it is not Me that is wrong. It's the way I've been taught to think about me and how to take care of me. By golly, we're going to figure it out."

In that moment, I had placed a metaphorical stake in the ground. I said to myself, "From this moment forward, I'm not going to listen to what my doctors are telling me, because they're not helping me. From this moment forward, I'm not going to believe them when they say I am going to get cancer. From this moment forward, I'm not going to believe them when they say I *need* the LEEP and vaccine. I'm not going to believe them when they try to push fear upon me so that I then comply with their treatments. No. No more. No more this way. I am taking back my power and I'm going to figure this out." And with that, I made a choice: *I was going to heal myself.*

In that moment, I had taken my power back, and empowered myself to move forward; to persevere and to figure out what was going on in my body. If Western medicine wasn't going to help me, then I was going to help myself.

Thus began my healing journey.

I began to look at the way I was living my life, and the way I was relating to my body. I began to notice all the ways in which I was not supportive of my body. I realized when I began this journey, I was diving into something so deep; so immense inside myself, that I wasn't sure whether I would come out the other side.

I completely overhauled my lifestyle. I stopped staying out late. I stopped drinking beer. I stopped going to pizza at 11 pm. I stopped hanging out with 'friends' who supported this unhealthy lifestyle. Yet most importantly, I stopped resisting myself. I stopped pushing down the Voice of my Body who for years, had been trying to tell me that something was wrong and that I needed to listen.

I learned about nutrition, beneficial herbs and supplements, habits that are helpful or detrimental to cervical health, spiritual practices, sexual practices, addressed how I was relating to and thinking about my body — I even started touching and loving my cervix just to connect (not for the purpose of pleasure). I began to spend more time in nature. I began to recognize how my own reproductive cycle and system actually mirrors and mimics that of the earth. I began to study indigenous ways of medicine and read stories about spontaneous healing. I even went back to school and received my Master of Arts in Integrative Health Studies, just so I could learn how human bodies heal and how we as driver of the human body can support in its healing.

I spent three long years researching and compiling all the information I could about the cervix and cervical dysplasia. I transformed my life to fit the needs of my body and my cervix, in order to support my body in doing what it does inherently — regenerate and heal.

Now, in all honesty, this was not an easy process for me. Throughout these three years, my pap tests remained abnormal. I still had HPV, and I still had cervical dysplasia, but I didn't let it bring me down. I continued to persevere. I continued to research. I continued to practice and integrate what I learned. I continued to study my body and my body's relationship to the world.

Over the course of those three years, there were dozens of times where I wanted to give up.

Every time my pap came back abnormal, I wanted to throw in the towel and resign to the fact that I'd be this way forever, or else I was going to get cancer. I would lament to my boyfriend how hopeless this process seemed — especially when the cervical dysplasia went up a grade. My Mother worried about me and continued to advise me to follow the doctor's orders — but no. I was committed, and going to see the process through.

On February 1st, 2015, I received a phone call that would change my life forever.

It was a Saturday afternoon when I heard my phone ring, showing me a number I didn't recognize. I answered anyway. My Nurse Practitioner greeted me on the other end. I thought it strange that she was calling me from her private line on a Saturday, and wondered if something was wrong. Normally, we had communicated through the office's online messaging platform.

She said, "Denell, I have something to tell you, and I couldn't wait to send you a message. Remember when you came in for a pap last week?"

"Well, yes, I remember. I come in pretty regularly. What's going on?" I asked.

"Well, I got your results back yesterday evening and they have been sitting with me... and I need to tell you something," she replied.

By this time, I was getting a little scared. I thought she was going to tell me that the cervical dysplasia had progressed even more and that I had cancer.

I was wrong.

She said, "Denell, you are clear. HPV is gone. You have no cervical dysplasia. In fact, your cervix is the healthiest I've ever seen it."

There was silence on the phone, as I sat in shock.

"Denell, how did you do it?!" she asked on the other line.

I burst out laughing as soon as she asked me that question.

This wasn't just any laugh, but a full-on witch's cackle; a howling laugh. One of complete excitement, jubilation and relief. I'd done it. I'd actually done it! *I Healed Myself.* Against all odds, against everything my doctors had told me; against everything Western medicine had said to me — the scare tactics, the bullying and shaming — I'd done it. Me and my body, together. **WE HAD HEALED.** I healed myself of cervical dysplasia and HPV after *seven years* of the same diagnosis. Seven years from the first diagnosis to that final phone call.

Little did I know that the phone call had also initiated me into a *new* journey.

On the one hand, I was so happy and excited that my cervix was clear and I didn't have to worry anymore about abnormal paps or colposcopies or cervical cancer or the LEEP. And on the other hand, the stark reality of the true situation hit me like a ton of bricks: There are *millions* of Women who have gone through (and continue to go through) the same exact experience as I had, complying with treatment plans they most likely don't understand, just as I didn't. There were women who didn't feel that pull towards putting a metaphorical stake in the ground, and followed through with what Western medicine requested of them. My heart sank realizing how little we Women are told about cervical health and the spark of activism ignited.

I was in my final semester of graduate school when I received the 'clear' test results I'd been waiting for. In one of my final classes, I was prompted to create a health education program about a disease or condition. I collected all the information I had discovered about the cervix, cervical dysplasia and HPV while healing and put it together into a presentation in celebration of my clear bill of health. I stood in front of the class, proudly sharing the sex education we'd never received with the women of my cohort, and they sat there listening to me, mouths agape.

Afterwards, several of them came up to me, asking, "Denell, why have you never talked about this before?"

"Well, I didn't really think about it. I didn't think anybody would want to hear about the cervix, or HPV. These are two topics that bring up a lot of shame and fear in people," I replied.

"Denell, you *must* talk about this. You *must* spread this information, because there are thousands, maybe even millions of women who deal with this, who are so scared, and feel like they can't talk about it with anyone," they said.

And so, here I am, telling you my story; talking about the cervix and cervical wellness. It took seven years from the time of my initial diagnosis to receiving that fateful phone call. It took over three years of concerted effort, trial and error in readapting lifestyle changes for me to *finally be clear.*

I share this with you, to tell you that it is possible. You don't have to have cervical dysplasia forever. Cervical dysplasia is, in fact, your body sending you a message, saying, "Hey! Hey! Over here! Look at me! I want to be looked at!"

As someone who has been through the healing journey, I know how scary it is. I know how utterly terrifying it is to receive these diagnoses. But, dear friend, *you can do this.* The only reason I can say this is, I have done it, myself.

There is so much we are not told about the cervix, including how to keep it healthy and well. Cervical Wellness, the project from which this book has been inspired by, emerged from the realization that there is a lack of information and *healing support* for the female reproductive system.

All people with cervixes need to know this information. This is truly the sex education we never received.

I am so happy and grateful to know that you are here, reading this book, learning about your cervix. This information will change your life forever, and will help change the course of Women's Health as we know it. It's about time women become thoroughly educated about their bodies, so that they can make informed and empowered choices for themselves.

The intention of this book is thus: To leave you feeling informed, aware and empowered when it comes to the health of your cervix, whether you're faced with an abnormal pap test result, or you use it as preventative medicine.

My hope is, by the end of this book, you will feel like you have the tools and resources you need to heal yourself, and to know in your heart that yes, you *can* heal yourself.

Thank you for being here. Thank you for saying YES to learning this information. Healing HPV and cervical dysplasia takes this sort of choice. You are either all in, or you are not. You are either committed to figuring your body out, or you are not. There is no halfway in healing.

Thank you for being willing to connect to your cervix.

This is the beginning of something amazing.

INTRODUCTION

Welcome to the incredible world of your *CERVIX*: The entryway to the center of your reproductive anatomy; the location in a female body where creativity, inner fire, and new life grow. The cervix is often overlooked when it comes to women's health, with most attention paid to the vagina, uterus, and ovaries. This is unfortunate, as the cervix is one of the most incredible aspects of the Female body.

It is the doorway for newborns to pass through as they enter this world, the energetic connector to Earth, and a place of potential, incredible pleasure. The cervix is a focal point of immunological health for the lower half of the body, the protector of the womb, the passageway for menstruation, the director of sperm for conception and holds the stories of our entire sexual history. When our cervix is healthy and we are connected to it, we can expect immense creative potential,

21

easeful gestation and birth (of babies or creative endeavors), immune vitality, and a deep connection to the Earth.

Join me on this journey to *explore the cervix*, and all the ways we can support its health and healing.

PART ONE | THE INFORMATION
THE SEX ED YOU NEVER RECEIVED

CHAPTER ONE
CERVIX, CERVICAL DYSPLASIA AND HPV

THE CERVIX

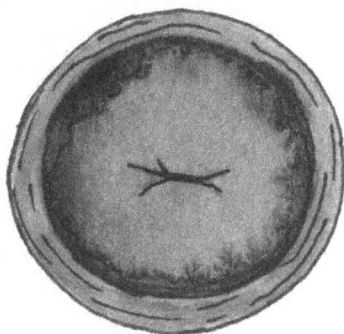

MY beautiful friends, welcome to **The Cervix**. The cervix is the tip of the uterus — also known as the 'neck' of the uterus — that rests gently between the vaginal canal and the uterus.

This is what the cervix looks like when viewed through the vaginal canal. The cervix is rounded, like a beautiful little mound, and protrudes ever-so-slightly into the vaginal canal. What we are looking at here is what is known as the 'face' of the cervix; that hole in the middle is called the cervical os, also known as the 'mouth'. What I find incredibly beautiful is how the cervix has a 'face' and a 'mouth' and is the 'neck' of the uterus. This essentially means it is another one of '*you*'; only, down below, in your lower half.

What we are looking at here is a vaginal canal that has been spread open, with the use of a speculum and a light. A light is needed to see the cervix because of how dark it is inside the vaginal canal. In this image, you can see the face, and the cervical os, as well as notice its natural roundness.

I believe it is so important to know exactly what you are working with when deepening your connection to heal your cervix of HPV and cervical dysplasia. It is very difficult to connect with something, when all you have ever seen of it is a clipart drawing of what it looks like, in 2D, and when you can, then, only roughly estimate as to where it is located inside the body. This is what you are working with to heal. Together, You (your ego / personality) and your Body will work together, in collaboration with this body part, in order to fully heal.

The face of the cervix can be pointed in various directions, depending on the time of the month and where you are in your fertility cycle. Sometimes, the cervical os is facing so far sideways that it looks like the cervix is hiding. This repositioning of the cervical face is perfectly normal.

I invite you to do web-search for photos of the cervix or head to the Beautiful Cervix Project web address found in the resource section. Take a moment to gaze upon an image of the cervix, and then to tune into your own body to connect to your own cervix, in knowing that this is what she looks like. I use the word 'She', but you can use whatever name or pronoun works for you.

ROLES OF THE CERVIX IN THE FEMALE BODY

THE roles of the Cervix in the female body are multifaceted, and encompass several aspects of female physiology.

In the most basic sense, the cervix is a portal. *Portal* is defined as an 'entrance or doorway', and that is exactly what the cervix is. It is the doorway between the outer world (the vaginal canal) and the inner world (the uterus) of a female body. The cervix is a portal to and from the womb. This doorway encompasses the entirety of the life-death-rebirth cycle contained within the female body.

Portal of Life

The cervical os is the doorway through which semen enters into the uterus, in order for conception to occur. When a penis enters into the vaginal canal, the head of the penis comes into contact with the face of the cervix. When ejaculation occurs, the ejaculate finds itself adjacent to the face of the cervix. Depending on where you are in the fertility cycle, the os of the cervix is either open or closed, and produces a variance of cervical fluid. The cervical fluid produced by the cervix mimics the consistency and pH of semen, thereby creating a 'ladder' for the sperm to swim up to enter into the doorway (the os). Once inside

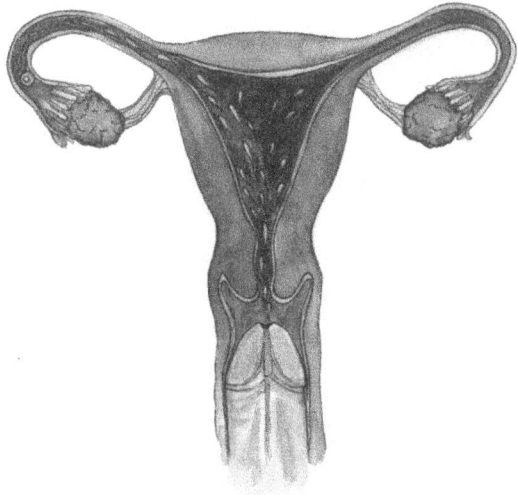

the doorway, the sperm can then make their way through the uterus and into the fallopian tubes, with the hope of fertilizing an ovulated egg.

Semen is not yet considered 'inside' of a female body until it enters into through cervical os. The vaginal canal, while it appears to be 'inside', is not actually considered a part of the internal viscera of female physiology. Given that the vaginal canal is like a collapsed tube, there really is no barrier between the inner vaginal canal and the outside world. If the cervical os is the doorway into the inner world of a female body, the vaginal canal serves as its entranceway. Hence, once semen passes through the cervical os (a doorway of Life), it then finds itself to be inside of the female body.

Portal of Birth

The most notable and obvious way in which the cervix is a portal for Life is in the birthing process of a physical baby. The cervix literally transforms itself into an open doorway so that the uterus can push the baby out through the use of contractions. The cervix effaces (becomes thinner) and the os dilates up to ten centimeters wide. The flexibility of the cervix allows for stretching to give way for the baby that's coming through.

The cervix is a literal threshold through which those who were born via vaginal birth passed. While in the uterus, the infant is still in the inner world of the Mother's body. Yet when it is time to be born into this physical world, the doorway opens and the child crosses through that threshold. The vaginal canal is akin to a building's hallway with an entrance leading to the outside world. The cervix is that doorway.

A teacher of mine once told me the story of the first birth she ever witnessed, and how she saw with her own eyes how the cervix is a portal. She said how, at the height of the labor experience — when the woman was dilated ten cm and amidst her final pushes — she had the opportunity to look into the woman's vaginal canal. My teacher said that what she saw forever changed her perspective on female reproductive anatomy.

What she saw was a dark, swirling, open portal. She is a Doctor of Indigenous Medicine and a Medical Intuitive, and as such, speaks of energy often. She told me how when she gazed into the birthing Woman's vaginal canal, it was like looking into a dark pool that was swirling. Like a scene from a science-fiction movie, a head appeared out of nowhere in this black vortex-like space. Suddenly, a whole baby emerged from this place and she wept at the beauty of what she witnessed. She told me, for the first time in her life, she understood how the cervix is a portal, and just how, through which, new human life is born.

Portal of Death

Having been a part of the Women's Wellness circle for a few years now, I've noticed a pattern within the offerings and figureheads of its field. Most education and support offered centers around birth, fertility and the beauty of feminine-Being. The female body is able to conceive, gestate and birth a brand-new human into this world, and the miracle of this is highly celebrated. I believe birth does need to be celebrated, and that the cervix, as this doorway through which life and birth occur, also needs to be celebrated. However, what I don't see in the Women's health field is support and celebration around the converse of birth and the portal of life: That is, honoring the cervix as a portal of death.

Western culture tends to turn a blind eye to death, keeping conversations to a minimum and hidden behind closed doors. Death and darkness tend to be perceived as 'bad' or 'evil', as we attempt to eliminate all notion of them from our daily lives. Regardless of this outrageous attempt at eliminating death, darkness and the shadow from our consciousness, millions of Women every year experience this darkened aspect of Womanhood in the form of menstruation, abortion and miscarriage. These experiences in which blood, tissue and life-matter flow out of the womb and through the cervix — not as life but as something that can no longer be life — characterizes the cervix as a portal of death.

Many people may be quick to assume that menstruation is not a 'death', yet when looking at the physiological standpoint of the natural process, it very much is a death, albeit a small one. Women are born with a finite amount of eggs within their ovaries. There are only so many fertility cycles a woman will go through before she no longer has any viable eggs and her body can no longer conceive a child. Unlike male bodies, female bodies have a start and end time to their fertility. Each cycle, one (or multiple) of these precious eggs are released from the ovary into the fallopian tube, in the hopes of being fertilized.

Regardless of whether the individual is mentally or emotionally prepared to conceive a child, the body is biologically primed to continue this process. When this precious egg is not fertilized and implanted, that life potential is lost forever. Two weeks after this missed conception,

31

the female body then sheds the uterine lining that could have supported this new life, and the uterine lining and accompanying blood flows out of the sacred doorway of the female reproductive system — the cervix.

The experiences of abortion and miscarriage fall along the same line, but are more intense in nature. Abortion is the choice of death: It is the conscious decision to end the life which is growing inside the womb of the body, and to bring about blood. This decision is the choice of the individual and it is alone her right to determine whether or not she wants to carry that life. This is the power that Women hold within them. The power to choose Life or to choose Death.

Miscarriage is on this same spectrum, only on the opposite side of abortion. It is the experience of losing a Life that was possibly desired, and experiencing this death; this loss within the body. This experience can be quite traumatic for the emotional body of the individual. To experience Death when Life was desired can invoke a deep period of grief that, for some Women, lasts a lifetime. I know many who have experienced miscarriages and pine for their would-be child, even years later.

In both these experiences, the cervix becomes the portal through which death emerges. In lieu of Life flowing through the portal, Death does. That which could have been life exits out the womb, through the cervix, and returns to Earth.

Many Women experience abortions and miscarriages in hospitals or in clinical settings, where they are unable to honor the life potential that had been carried within them. The blood of the death is lost to hazardous waste dump sites and sanitary cleaners. The blood is unable to return to the Earth, where it can then be reintegrated into Earth's ecosystem. I believe that this dishonoring on the part of the Western medical establishment only increases the prevalence of mental unwellness, regret, and shame surrounding these experiences with death.

I wonder what it would be like for Women to bury their aborted or miscarried child in the Earth through ceremony. What would it be like for Women to sit on the Earth while they bled and watched as it's reabsorbed into the Earth? I wonder what it would be like for Women to be honored for being a carrier of the Portal of Death, rather than be shamed or made to feel guilty for it?

There is a movement amongst Women to give their menstrual blood back to the Earth. I know many Women in the birth and reproductive wellness world who invite their clients and social media followers to collect their menstrual blood via menstrual cups or cloth pads rinsed in water (the water collected) to be given as offerings to plants and to the Earth. It is known through organic gardening practices that plants thrive on blood and bone fertilizer, and our own blood is no different. Plants thrive when given these offerings. More and more women are setting aside time to be in nature, to sit with their yonis open to the Earth, as they allow the blood to flow freely through the cervix straight into the soil, grass or moss below.

What if we took this one step further and offered all our blood — *all* of the reality of being carriers of the Portal of Death — to the Earth? How would that change the way abortion and miscarriage are considered throughout Western society? How would that change the way Women are treated during these times of loss, when they are so enveloped in the shroud of death?

Connection to the cervix as a portal of death is equally as important as connection to it as a portal of life. The cervix holds the keys to this connection. Which way are we headed? Toward the continued dishonoring of the death that has exited a Woman's body? Or, on the contrary, closer to a paradigm in which we remember the beauty of Death, and allow that potential of what could have been to return to where it originated... the Earth? I believe it's high time the cervix and Women's experiences of death within their bodies are

33

honored and treated as sacred. Imagine a world where women gather to give their loss to the Earth, transmuting something once ignored amidst society into something revered and approached with respect to its essence.

This is how we can honor the cervix as this sacred portal. This is how we can honor the Sacred Anatomy of the Female Body. This is how we can remember these hallowed experiences of Womanhood.

Portal of Pleasure

One of the many miracles of this body part is the cervical orgasm! I have heard cervical orgasms are the ultimate state of bliss a Woman can experience. Teachers of Tantra, and other sacred sexual practices, speak to the power of cervical orgasms and how they can leave a Woman in a blissful state for hours or even days. The cervix is the site of potential incredible pleasure! Unfortunately, this is not spoken of often.

Cervical orgasms are different than clitoral and g-spot orgasms. They do not follow the same arc of experience. Clitoral orgasms tend to stimulate male orgasm. There is a buildup, a peak experience, and then a release. In cervical orgasm, there is no 'end'.

Kim Anami, tantra and sacred sexuality teacher, says the process of a cervical orgasm follows more of a build-up of pleasure, plateau, build-up of pleasure, plateau, build-up of pleasure, plateau type of experience. Unlike in a clitoral orgasm, where there is a release and a decrease of energy, cervical orgasms build up energy that remains at that level in the female body system.

Many Women who have experienced cervical orgasm speak to its potential in feeling like a 'spiritual experience'. There is such an opening of energy and pleasure within the body that the mind quiets completely, leaving the individual completely immersed in the experience of the pleasure of their body.

Dr. Barry Komisaruk, psychological professor and researcher at Rutgers University, mapped how the physical sensation of pleasure from the cervix is communicated to the brain. He found that the cervix has more nerve pathways than any other part of the female sexual anatomy. The four nerve pathways which connect the cervix to the brain are the vagus, hypogastric, and pelvic. The cervix is primed to be one of the most pleasurable places within the female body. There's a movement made by the cervix called the 'cervical kiss' where, through the right stimulation and within the context of safety, the cervix appears to move downward into the vaginal canal and expand open. This is the cervix opening and readying itself to become the portal of pleasure.

In order for a cervical orgasm to be achieved, a Woman must be open, connected and in touch with her body during the sexual experience. If a Woman is in her mind, worrying about something or fearful in anyway, she will not be able to reach cervical orgasm. Relaxation and a sense of safety is key to tune into those nerve pathways. Mental and emotional preparation is necessary for cervical pleasure; one must be 'dropped into' the cervix and be willing to surrender to the experience.

The cervix must also be in the correct physical position (high in the vaginal canal). When it isn't, the cervix can experience pain during penetration. Very often, Women shut down physically during sex because they feel pain in their cervix, and this then prevents them from experiencing pleasure there. Unfortunately, this is an all too common experience for many Women. It is said that under 10% of Women experience pleasure and orgasm in their cervix.

Cervix, Sex and Position

In everyday living, the cervix sits rather low in the vaginal canal; anywhere between two to four inches above the vaginal opening. Throughout the duration of the fertility cycle this is in flux, but in general when a Woman is *not* sexually aroused, the cervix is positioned rather low in the vaginal canal.

The cervix is intelligent: She knows what's up. When you become sexually aroused, the cervix receives the 'message' that something may soon be entering into the vaginal canal through a cascade of hormones that are initiated with arousal. The cervix does not want to get hit or damaged from whatever may penetrate the vaginal canal, so what does she do? She moves upward into the body cavity via a movement of the uterus, and thus out of the way. The cervix *literally* moves up into the body to create more space in the vaginal canal in preparation for penetration. Six to eight inches of space is created through this movement, tucking the cervix away, safe from physical harm. The cervix places itself at the proper distance for stimulation as she takes on her role as a portal for pleasure. The uterus also tilts backwards, aiding the cervix in protecting its face.

Female bodies need more time to 'warm up' for sex not because we are stiff or controlling; rather, it is for the physical safety of our bodies. When time is not given for the female body to prepare for penetration, the cervix feels the dull pain of being 'hit'. Almost every Woman I speak to can relate to that sensation of 'thumping' (the sharp internal pain of being penetrated too deeply). I've also heard men say they 'hit her back' or have 'bottomed-out'. No, it is not the 'back' or 'bottom'. It is the cervix, and it hurts. That pain, which so many Women feel during sex, is the voice of the cervix saying "I'm not quite into position yet, and am not ready for penetration. A little more time would be helpful!"

36

Next time you are about to engage in sex, and you are not fully aroused, remember the voice of your cervix. Use your own voice to speak up for her when you feel her pain. Remember, it is *your* body and *you* get to decide who/what penetrates you in *your* own time. Not your partner's, nor anyone else's.

I invite you to take a moment and ask yourself:

"Am I connected to my cervix?"

"Have I ever felt pleasure in my cervix?"

"How can I deepen my relationship with my cervix so I *can* feel pleasure?"

"What would it be like if I was not only connected to my cervix, but felt its pleasure too?"

"What is preventing or blocking me from connecting with my cervix to feel pleasure?"

Grab a journal and answer these questions. You may be surprised by the answers that arise.

CERVICAL DYSPLASIA

THE Cervix is a resilient and strong organ, holding the roles as a portal of pleasure, birth and death. Yet regardless of the amazing potential of power residing within it, the cervix is highly sensitive and vulnerable, too. This vulnerable, sensitive nature causes the cervix to play focal point in gynecological exams, and it is suggested by Allopathic medicine that all females have pap-smears to monitor its health.

Pap-smears take small, superficial cell-samples from the face of the cervix to check the health of the cells located there. When these tests come back showing signs of 'abnormality', the diagnosis of 'cervical dysplasia' is then given.

Cervical dysplasia is a really fancy way of saying 'abnormal cells on the cervix'. Even though this phrase is quite simple, questions such as 'what does abnormal mean?', 'what is actually wrong?', and 'how did this happen?' naturally arise.

Cervical dysplasia arises on the face of the cervix — the exposed portion of the cervix within the vaginal canal. This portion of the cervix is unique from the rest of the uterine body, in that it has a special section of cells called the squamocolumnar junction, or 'the transformation zone'. It is in this location that cervical dysplasia arises.

The squamocolumnar junction is the location on the face of the cervix where one type of cell transforms into another type of cell — hence the name 'transformation zone'. The cells from the interior of the cervical os (columnar cells) move and travel from the inside of the cervical canal/os and become a part of the face of the cervix (squamous cells). The location where the columnar cells transform into squamous cells is the 'squamocolumnar junction', or more colloquially, 'the transformation zone'.

Our cervix produces new cells every day. Just like every other

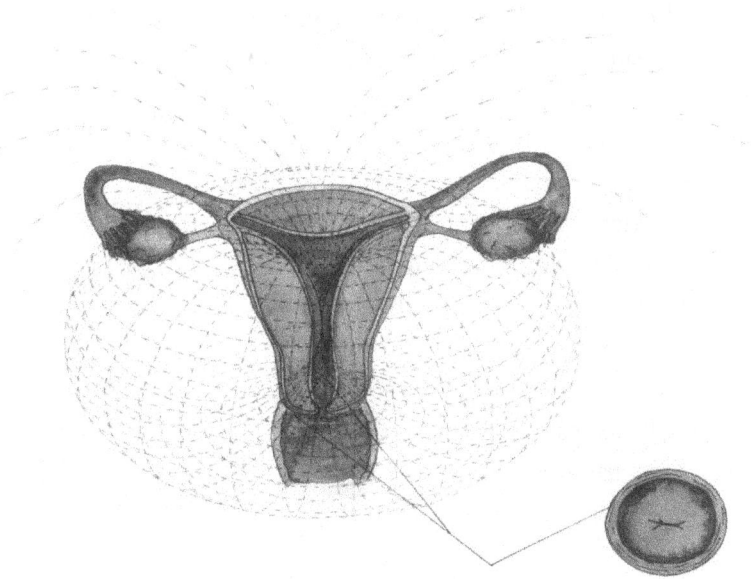

portion of our body, the cells of the cervix regenerate in order to keep us healthy and well. The cervix regenerates in a manner that can be best described by looking at an image of a torus.

Just as a torus flows upward and out in a continuous fashion, so do the regenerating cells of the cervix. All the cells in the center of the cervical os eventually travel to become the cells of the face. The long, skinny columnar cells of the cervical canal and os make their way to the face, change shape, and become short, fat squamous cells.

Cervical dysplasia is found in the transformation zone and within the cervical canal (inside the os). Dysplastic cells can be understood to be cells that are not 'transforming' in a healthy way and become 'abnormal'. This can be likened to how a caterpillar transforms into a butterfly. In that in-between state of metamorphosis, the cells and body of the transforming caterpillar are extremely delicate. This is also true for the cells of the transformation zone of the cervix. These cells around the outside of the cervical os are very sensitive and vulnerable. When the cervix is not taken care of, and the cells continue to transform abnormally, cervical cancer may develop.

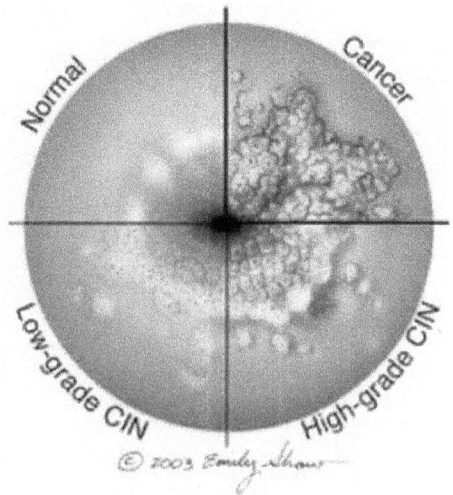

It is important to note that the cells of the transformation zone are also the most exposed portion of the cervix itself. These cells on the cervix's face are most susceptible to injury from sex or forceful penetration.

The process of fully healing the cervix of cervical dysplasia boils down to supporting the healthy regeneration of cells as they move through the transformation zone. We want to support the cervix in such a way that healthy transformation occurs as those new columnar cells are formed in the canal and make their way to the face.

This process takes time, as it is necessary for the older, abnormal cells to go through their lifecycle and become reabsorbed by the body.

Healing cervical dysplasia boils down to allowing the older, dysplastic cells to be replaced with new, healthy cells.

A Note About Pap-Smears

Pap-smears (pap tests) monitor this special transformation zone to ensure the cells are transforming in a healthy way. The whole point of a pap smear is to see how those columnar cells are changing into squamous cells. The test checks the inside of the cervical canal and just outside the cervical os. How are these cells changing shape? Are they okay? This is the point of the pap smear.

The Pap test has saved millions of Women's lives worldwide. While paps are neither comfortable nor pleasurable, it is important we get our cervix checked, given that we cannot feel whether or not the cells are abnormal. These tests are a *lifesaver* for many, and a test that we here at Cervical Wellness recommend all those with female anatomy to receive. I would like to take a moment to honor the history of this test and briefly share its origin story.

Dr. Papanicolaou

Cervical cancer was one of the leading causes of death amongst women at the turn of the twentieth century. In an attempt to figure out a way to prevent premature death among reproductive-age women, Dr. George N. Papanicolaou researched ways to screen for precancerous conditions. Papanicolaou, a Greek pioneer in cytopathology and early cancer detection, published the now famous, "Diagnosis of Uterine Cancer by the Vaginal Smear" in 1943, and thus, the diagnostic procedure named the Pap-test was introduced to the Western medical field.[1]

ABNORMAL PAP TEST RESULTS

WHAT does it mean when your pap test results come back abnormal?

It means that the cells in the transformation zone of your cervix are not changing shape in the healthiest way and that there are signs of 'cervical dysplasia'. Cervical Dysplasia simply means, 'abnormal cells on the cervix'.

One word doctors like to throw into the mix when discussing abnormal pap test results is the big 'C' word — cancer. The use of this word causes profound distress for many Women, as it can feel like a death sentence when used in discussing one's cervical health. I am here to dispel the myth that just because you have abnormal cells on your cervix means that you are on track to develop cancer. While the abnormal cells on your cervix are an indication as such, the likelihood of your developing cervical cancer is relatively low.

The amount of time between first signs of abnormality on the cervix to the development of full-blown cancer can range anywhere between 10-25 years.[2] Cervical cancer will arise if you choose to ignore your results and to not do anything about your health situation. Even then, it may take up to a decade to fully develop.

The truth is that our bodies are always producing cancerous cells. Cancer is, simply put, your own cells in your body mutating and becoming abnormal. I actually have a big problem with the phrase 'war against cancer' because this literally means a 'war against your own body' or a 'war against yourself'. You are fighting your own body.

Regardless of this nuance of words, it is important to know that when these cells are abnormal and not listened to (see the Voice of the Body section), that they can then develop into cancer.

Cervical Wellness teaches that anything 'wrong' in the body (such as these abnormal cells) is a message from your body (and your cervix) that needs to be listened to. Something you are doing on behalf of your body is not working. The only way our bodies can tell us something isn't working is by producing these abnormal cells. So many of us are numbed to the feelings and sensations of our bodies, and very often we ignore or don't realize there is a message being sent to us. Sometimes we receive the messages and then don't believe them or chalk it up to it 'being all in our head'. Due to this ignorance and disbelief, the body does what it knows how to do, and that is to change itself. It starts producing cells in the transformation zone that are abnormal so that you bring your attention there.

When we decide not to listen and ignore this message from our body, our body gets upset. The message becomes louder. This is when the cervical dysplasia increases in severity. When the message is still ignored, the body goes into 'last hope' mode. The body begins to yell and scream. This is when cancer develops. *Our body does not want to die*, and will do everything in its power to send you the message that something needs to change.

Having abnormal cells on the cervix doesn't mean that our body is against us. *The abnormality is actually our body trying to get our attention.* Our body longs for us to be in partnership and connection with it so that we (the 'I' that is your ego plus your body) can be healthy and well. When

43

we don't listen, our body will continue to get sick, and we may die —
which is the last thing our body wants. Our body desires wholeness; our
natural state is one of health and constructive growth.

The abnormal cells on your cervix are a message that you need
to bring some attention and love to this place in your body. An
abnormal pap means it is time to give your cervix some love and
attention, which is actually an amazing opportunity to connect to a place
within you that perhaps you have never connected to before.

HPV

ONE of the most widely known causes of cervical dysplasia is the human papillomavirus or HPV. The diagnosis of cervical dysplasia quite often comes in tandem with the diagnosis of HPV.

HPV is transmitted through intimate skin-to-skin contact, primarily during sexual intercourse. It is the most commonly known sexually transmitted infection (STI) and "is so common that nearly all sexually active men and women get it at some point in their lives."[3] The human immune system generally combats the virus before any signs or symptoms can occur and most people will never know they even had it. According to the Center for Disease Control "HPV can be passed even when an infected person has no signs or symptoms. You can develop symptoms years after you have sex with someone who is infected, making it hard to know when you first became infected." [4]

As of 2010, roughly 79 million sexually active adults in the United States have been infected with some strain of the HPV virus, and what with the advent of family-planning options that do not require the need for barrier protection, it seems as though these numbers are rising.[5]

It is amidst the innocence of discovering new sexual partners that this STI gets passed from individual to individual, hanging around like a silent hitchhiker looking for the next ride. Many women who are on hormonal contraceptives tend to believe there's nothing to worry about, and thus allow unprotected sexual penetration. If they do not routinely get tested for HPV infection, they may never know they have it, which then increases their risk of developing cervical dysplasia.

There are risk factors associated with sexual intercourse that can cause cervical cells to become abnormal and precancerous in women. The first major risk factor for women is becoming sexually active before the age of twenty. This is because the squamo-cellular junction (the area of the cervix that becomes abnormal) moves upwards into the endocervical canal with age, yet in younger women these cells are exposed, making them more vulnerable to infection.[6] Another risk factor is having multiple sex partners or having a partner who themselves has multiple partners, which simply heightens potential exposure to HPV.[7] This reality is only exacerbated by the increased sexualization of children and teens in mass media. Cultural norms subvertly pressure young adults to engage in sexual activity at an early age, putting young women at risk for STIs such as HPV.

Some other interesting information about HPV that is not widely known:

- There are 118 strains of HPV
- 40 infect the throat, vaginal canal, anal canal, and cervix
- 5 strains of HPV lead to cancer
- The HPV vaccine 'Gardasil 9' targets four of them
- Can be passed from male -> female without knowledge

Regardless of the prevalence of HPV, many people engage in unprotected sex. This, coupled with high-stress lifestyles, leaves the immune system vulnerable to viral infection. Lifestyles which include late-night partying, multiple sex partners, and ignorance towards female reproductive health concerns leave many Women unknowingly at risk for contracting the virus and developing cervical dysplasia.

A Note About the HPV-Vaccine

For the sake of keeping this book helpful and light-hearted, I've largely left out my opinion and thoughts on the HPV vaccine. In short, I neither support nor advocate for the vaccine in my work with Cervical Wellness.

The research I've done on vaccine injury due to Gardasil is scary and overwhelming, to say the least. If you or someone you love is considering opting in for Gardasil or any other HPV vaccine, I invite you to 1) read the information-insert that comes in the box with the vaccine *in full* (you can request this from your doctor), 2) do your own research about the side-effects and injury reports from the vaccine, 3) research the statistics of cervical cancer deaths vs. Gardasil vaccine injury deaths and determine which is the greater risk, and 4) trust your gut.

Vaccines are a modern-marvel and important to use in certain viral/bacterial cases (like smallpox, malaria, yellow fever, etc.). However, I do question the use of a vaccine-series for a virus that's been deemed 'the common cold of the cervix' and can quite easily be reversed through lifestyle intervention.

I am not telling you to not get the vaccine. What I am saying is to do your own due diligence and to research (for more than 10 minutes on the internet) before saying yes. This way, you will be informed, aware, and empowered in your decision.

HOW TO PREVENT HPV
FLARE-UP

Hpv is a virus, just like the common cold or the flu. Whether or not a virus overtakes a human body is determined by the state of an individual's immune system. Viruses work by injecting their genetic makeup into a person's cells, causing the cellular function of the individual to act in favor of multiplying viral bodies throughout the system. A more technical explanation is as follows:

Viruses exploit the 'machinery' of human cells by producing proteins which the virus needs in order to replicate. The virus penetrates into the host cell where it then injects its RNA, the copy of its DNA, into the cell. RNA is considered a 'cookbook' containing the recipe of proteins the virus needs for its replication. Each cell in the body has ribosomes, which move along the RNA, reading the code for the proteins that need to be produced in order to fulfill the needs of the cell. Viruses are tricky, in that their RNA are similar to that of the host cell's, and as such, the ribosomes will start reading the viral RNA to produce proteins for the virus without question. Essentially, the virus is like a parasite, exploiting the human cell in order to live and reproduce.[8]

The immune system is what fights off and curtails the virus' efforts to inject its RNA into the body's host cells. I like to think of the immune system as our protector. It surveys the body, seeking and destroying any invaders encountered in the system, like a virus.

The Immune System

The human immune system is an intricate network of organs that work in tandem to ward off invaders. Organs that constitute the immune system include the tonsils and adenoids, lymph nodes and lymphatic vessels, thymus, spleen, and bone marrow. Each place in the body serves a different function for the immune system. Each must be healthy in order for the immune system to function properly. If one place in the system is not operating smoothly, the entire mechanism hiccups. In order to function properly, this defense system must be able to detect a wide variety of pathogens and distinguish them from the host's own healthy tissue.

The immune system can be broken down into two subsystems — the innate immune system and adaptive immune system.

The innate immune system is the body's first line of defense.

When pathogens enter the body, they encounter the cells and mechanisms of this system. Aspects of the innate immune system include:

- Surface barriers (mucous membranes, gastric acid, vaginal secretions, skin, etc.) and their mechanisms (coughing, sneezing, urination, vomiting)
- Inflammation (which increases blood flow and increases cytotoxic [cell-killing] factors which recruit immune cells to the site of infection)
- The complement systems (a biochemical cascade attacking the surfaces of foreign cells)

49

- Cellular barriers, such as leukocytes (white blood cells) which identify and eliminate pathogens in the blood system
- Natural killer cells (which destroy compromised host cells).

The adaptive immune system, on the other hand, allows for a stronger immune response and immunological memory, where each pathogen is 'remembered' by a specific antigen. An antigen is a molecule capable of inducing an immune response to produce an antibody. This branch of the immune system is antigen specific. This means that there must be recognition of 'non-self' in order for the process of adaptive immunity to be initiated, wherein antibodies are produced to fight off the pathogen.

Aspects of adaptive immunity include:

- Lymphocytes (special white blood cells which include B cells and T cells and are created in the bone marrow)
- Killer T cells (a subgroup of T cells that kill cells infected with a virus)
- Helper T cells (which regulate both adaptive and innate immune responses to help determine which response to activate)
- Other B cells and antibodies.

Each T cell and B cell recognizes different antigens which have been memorized through immunological memory.

Immunological memory occurs when B cells and T cells have been activated and replicated. The 'offspring' of these originally activated cells become long-lived memory cells. Throughout the lifetime of a person, these memory cells remember each specific pathogen encountered and can initiate a stronger response if the pathogen is detected again.

As you can see, the human immune system is an intricate network of organs and cells which must work in tandem and cooperation to prevent the body from being overtaken by a pathogen. All aspects of the immune system are important in keeping the body healthy.

HPV and the Immune System

The human immune system generally fights off the HPV virus before any signs or symptoms occur, and most people will never know they had it. As mentioned previously, HPV can be passed even when an infected person has no signs or symptoms.

The key to preventing HPV from flaring up in your body is by keeping your immune system healthy and strong. When the immune system is strong, it will be able to stave off the HPV virus from taking root in your cells and flaring up in your body. You can be exposed to the virus, but it will not overtake your system.

Many Women experience a flare-up of HPV during a time in their lives where it is seemingly impossible to have contracted it. Sometimes they will be diagnosed with HPV when they're in a long-term partnership, and out of nowhere the HPV manifests. This can occur when exposure to the virus has happened in the past and circumstances in life have led the immune system to weaken, creating space for the virus to proliferate.

Some life experiences which may cause this to happen are:

- Another bacterial/viral infection
- High-stress experiences
- A sudden death or immense grief
- Another health concern

51

- Sudden life change

The first thing I inquire about is life circumstances when working with someone who's received an HPV diagnosis, and who's had the same sexual partner for several years. More often than not, the client has had either a) another viral or bacterial illness which weakened their immune system, or b) an extremely stressful life event. Both of these situations can hamper the functioning of your immune system and allow for the lurking HPV virus to find wiggle room and proliferate. If this is you, it's okay. You've done nothing wrong. Even if you're not in a long-term partnership and HPV has suddenly revealed itself in your life, you've done nothing wrong.

I want to remind you to be kind and compassionate to yourself if you have been diagnosed with HPV. The stresses of life, coupled with lack of information and awareness of this STI, have brought you to this point, but you can now make new and informed decisions for the love and support of your cervix, your reproductive system, and your whole body.

CHAPTER TWO
HOW TO HEAL

The trick to Cervical Self Care is simple: Engage in a lifestyle and daily habits that support your immune system and your body's natural ability to heal.

HEALING VS TREATMENT

SELF-HEALING and regeneration are what our body does naturally and inherently. It is always moving towards a state of health, wellness and wholeness. You know how you can cut off the tip of your finger and it will fully grow back, nail and all? Or how 75% of your liver can be removed, and yet it will fully regenerate to its original size within just a few months? This is true for all organs of our body, even the reproductive system. Our cervix is constantly growing new cells, working towards eliminating the ones which are not healthy. Our bodies are truly miraculous.

The process of healing can be a long one. There is a reason why I call it the 'healing journey'. It is a journey you take yourself on in order to bring about complete transformation, from the inside out. The process is one of excavating through the muck of your inner world to find the source of the pollutant — the reason(s) why you aren't getting better.

One thing doctors often don't tell their patients is that it takes time to heal. Not treatments, not a drug. *Time*. This notion of not having an immediate and quick fix goes against our Western cultural value of immediate and instant gratification, but this is the truth.

The process of actually healing yourself from whatever ails you, especially HPV and Cervical Dysplasia, happens from the inside out.

There is nothing someone else can do for you to help you heal. You must make the empowered decision to take the steps necessary to bring your body to a place where it can regenerate — which your body inherently knows how to do.

On Treatment

Western medicine is wonderful for certain things. I am so grateful for the availability of care for acute situations like a heart attack or stroke, for trauma care in the case of a severed limb or a wound needing stitches, and for the ability to test for and diagnose diseases and conditions. Allopathic medicine is wonderful at providing information and for taking care of crises relating to the body. Unfortunately, it is not very good at helping people to heal, especially chronic conditions that are caused by one's lifestyle.

Did you know most medical doctors receive less than five hours of instruction on nutrition? How could this be? If these individuals are trained to take care of our bodies, and we are made to believe they are there to support us in getting well, how can we trust in their ability to help us if they don't know the proper way to care for a body *before* something goes wrong?

Allopathic medicine is based upon a reductionist view of the body. This theory follows the understanding that the most complicated and complex systems can be explained by analyzing the simplest and most basic physical aspects of that system. The reductionist view of the human body looks at a single organ or aspect of an organ and sees it as a single individual, separate from the whole. Practitioners of allopathic medicine treat that single, individual part and trust everything else will be fine. The reason they see the body in this way is because the development of allopathic practices stems from research performed on cadavers, where the intricate vital life-force connecting all organs is no longer present. But this is, unfortunately, just not how the living human body works.

The human body is a highly complex biological system, with each organ system intricately linked to every other organ system. There is no beginning and no end within the human body. There is neither separation nor isolation of its moving parts. Each system affects one another. If something is wrong in one, it is highly likely there is something wrong in another.

Western medicine has led us to believe that the only way we can help ourselves is by allowing medical practitioners to 'treat' us. Western medicine is not in the business of healing; it is in the business of *treatment*. Truthfully, however; these treatments often tend to do more harm than good to our bodies.

It's well documented throughout non-Western medical models (i.e. Ayurveda and Traditional Chinese Medicine) that all parts of our body are interconnected and communicate with one-another, whereas Western mindsets have been trained to see the human body from a reductionist viewpoint — that analyzing the simplest part and offering treatment thereof, will fix whatever is wrong. Regardless of whatever viewpoint we are looking from, what we know about the human body is limited to how we have developed our language around it. If our medical practitioners see the body in this reductionist way, then they will treat it in that manner; meaning, by looking at just a single part regardless of what the whole is presenting.

Here is the definition of *Treatment*: *1 — The management or care of a patient, 2 — The combating of a disease or disorder.*

In no part of this definition does the word 'heal' or 'healing' occur. Treatment is about addressing the symptoms: The physical manifestations of an underlying root cause. Treatment is about 'combat'; about 'fighting a war against' and about the dissociation from the interconnection of all parts of the body.

56

Treatments focus solely on a single organ system, or even more commonly, a single organ or part of an organ. This disregards the fact that when there is un-wellness in one place in the body, then there is likely un-wellness in other places of the body as well. Treating the single organ or organ system is basically like putting a bandage on a deep wound or sliver, without actually cleaning the wound or removing the sliver. Treatments tend to be temporary fixes without long term gains. Most often, an individual will have to return to the doctor for more treatments, again and again, which facilitate a false sense of wellness without ever addressing the root cause of the dis-ease (disease meaning merely 'a lack of ease'). Often the condition returns, and the person will need to start another round of treatment.

In short, treatments do very little to help a person heal.

On Healing

Healing is the step beyond treatment and is the ultimate goal. Healing is the process of moving beyond what is ailing you, so you never have to worry about it or be treated for it ever again. Ever. Healing is wholeness.

The definition of *Healing: (literally meaning to make whole) is the process of the restoration of health from an unbalanced, diseased or damaged organism. The result of healing can be a cure to a health challenge, but one can heal without being cured.*

Cured is a word associated with treatment. As the definition states, one can heal without being cured.

In looking at this definition in comparison to the definition of treatment, the one thing that stands out to me most is this: **the restoration of health vs. combating of a disease**. The focus of treatment is on the disease or condition, and all attention is given to that which is 'wrong'. Whereas in healing, the attention is placed on balance

57

and wholeness; on restoration and regeneration. As the saying goes, 'That which you focus on, grows'. What do you want to grow more of? Disease and unwellness? Treatment and patient care? Or would you rather grow more of health and wellness; feeling good and thriving? This is an important distinction to make. Healing is the process of bringing back balance to the body system from the inside out. It is the uncovering of the message your body has been trying to send to you for who knows how long.

Did you know that your body has a voice? I know, sounds crazy right? But it does. Your body has a voice just like your mind has a voice; it's just quieter and more subtle than the voice of your mind. The voice of your mind is your inner dialogue, which speaks to you in thoughts and words. Most of us live by listening to the voice of our mind. Yet, for the next few minutes, I invite you to open up your perspective to include the notion that yes, your body, too, has a voice, and she has been waiting for you to hear her.

Voice of the Body

Imagine, for a moment, your body as a small child. You care for this small child by feeding it, keeping it safe and overall taking care for the health and life of this child. You are its keeper, and in essence, its parent.

Now imagine this small child gets an 'owie' or a wound of some kind. This wound can be physical (like having too much sugar in the blood or getting some sort of viral/bacterial infection) or this wound can be emotional (like experiencing a trauma, heartbreak, or abuse). This child will tell you when this wound occurs, and will communicate to you via the only way it knows — through emotions and showing something is 'wrong' so that you'll pay attention to it.

When something is 'wrong' in your body, it's actually your body sending you a message. The message is 'HEY look over here! Something is wrong and I'm unable to do what I'm supposed to do! Help me please!'. This 'wrong' thing is actually your body's voice crying out for attention and love. Anything 'abnormal' or 'out of balance' is your body wanting to send you a message that you haven't been taking care of it in the way it needs, and so it tries to communicate that to you.

Unfortunately, many of the treatments provided by Western medicine cut away this message, essentially silencing your body's attempt to cry for help. This then leads the 'wrong' to return, and sometimes worsen. The 'wrong' may come back with a vengeance, so you will actually pay attention this time. This is the child screaming and kicking, wanting you to hear and see it; to witness its pain and provide support.

The caveat to healing via listening to the voice of your body is that it takes *time* — sometimes longer than we're comfortable with. More often than not, fear takes over and we jump on the first option given, which leads to the silencing of our body at the hands of someone who isn't living in our body like we are and doesn't experience firsthand this message that's trying to come through.

In order to heal HPV and cervical dysplasia, you must take into account the messages your body is sending to you. These diagnoses are your body's way of calling your attention to this place, as it has a message for you waiting there. There is something inside you needing to be seen, expressed, listened to and integrated. Something is asking for you to notice it and love it and take care of it, like a small child in a tantrum, wanting your attention.

So, how do we heal?

HABIT CHANGE AND LIFESTYLE TRANSFORMATION

Change your habits, change your life.
The power of choice lies in your hands.

Habits are what direct us in daily living. They're the actions that we unconsciously take as we move through our day. Our habits determine how we feel about ourselves and how we portray ourselves in the world. Habits can lead you to a place of personal empowerment in health. Habits can lead you to great wealth and abundance. Habits can also lead you to disease and illness, or to financial hardship. Habits can, also, lead you to become disconnected from your own body and inner voice.

What's amazing about habits is that we have the power to change them in any moment. We have the capability to shift our habits to create the life we dream of and desire. If you want a strong body but are not achieving this, it is your habits with food and exercise that prevent you from reaching your goals. If you want financial freedom, it is your habits of making, spending and tracking your money that are preventing you from achieving this.

If you want to heal yourself of HPV and cervical dysplasia, you need to change your lifestyle and habits to meet the needs of your body and immune system. When you change your habits and actively work on them, your life will begin to transform.

The process of habit and lifestyle change is not linear: Meaning, you don't decide something is going to happen and then move through a step-by-step process to reach that goal wherein you are forever changed. In fact, it is quite the opposite.

Habit change moves you through a spiraling cycle that begins to ingrain a new habit or way of living into your psyche and consciousness. You must work to forge new neural pathways, because your old habits are already ingrained in your brain. One example of an ingrained habit is waking up in the morning and automatically putting milk and sugar in your coffee. It's how you've done it for years. It is ingrained in your neural network and you don't even think twice about doing it. Those neural pathways are very deeply carved into your mind.

The trick of habit formation is to recognize what you want to change, and then make a daily effort to forge new pathways. This all takes perseverance and doesn't happen overnight.

Perseverance isn't widely discussed in our instant-gratification culture. Many people begin a habit change — like changing a diet, or introducing a new exercise regimen — and give up when it starts to get difficult. The truth is that yes, there will be days (maybe most of them) where you don't want to engage this new habit. It is easier to just eat the same thing you've always eaten, or to not exercise because that is what you have always done. Yet if you continue on and persevere, eventually this new way of being will become equally as strong as your old way of doing things. Eventually, this new habit will become more deeply ingrained than the original one. One day you'll find yourself remembering how you used to live your life in that way, and you couldn't even imagine going back.

When you change your habits, you change your life. Quick fixes like treatment and surgeries are bandages that cover up the underlying problem of unhealthy habits.

This is *how* you change your life to heal: Through changing your lifestyle and your belief system surrounding your ability to do so.

Habits as Moments Spent in Time

Some of you may ask, why are you talking so much about habits? Why are you so passionate about habit formation? What drives me to spend a lot of time thinking about my habits is the understanding that habits are the ways we choose to *spend our time*. The key word here being *time*.

The reality is that our time on this planet, in this life, is finite. It isn't endless. It will not go on forever, and is in fact limited. We are all going to die someday. This truth leads me to consider how I want to fill my time. To me, time is the ultimate consideration. Although it can be argued that there is no such thing as time, that there is only this moment *right now*, the stark reality is that there won't always be a *now* in this body. I have come to terms with this and it is what propels me to be living in a way where I continuously say to myself, "Hey, this can end at any moment, and I want to think, do and be in the ways that make me feel the best I can! I want to be the best version of myself. Because why the heck not?"

Yes, you can choose to go in the opposite direction, and choose to be a version of yourself that perhaps doesn't highlight your most amazing qualities. And that is okay, because you get to choose. That is what is awesome about being a human.

However, you *can* choose to feel great and amazing in your body, in your life, and in your spirit. Anyone can. There is nothing that makes

62

me or anyone else who is living their best life more special or unique than you. You have all the capabilities as anyone else. It all boils down to how you want to spend your time with the habits that you have.

A Few More Thoughts on Habits

I do not buy into lifestyle transformation programs that say "Pay 39.99 and transform your body in 30 days with this video series" because what I know to be true is as soon as that month video series is over, the individual is most likely to go back to doing what they were doing beforehand. That pointed experience of 30 days of action will be great, but it will most likely not continue on. While this might seem pessimistic to point out, it is what I have observed in myself and many people in my life.

After nine years of habit change exploration and practice, I have come to determine a couple of things that are very important to take into consideration:

1.   Formation of a new habit is an act of devotion. It is a spiritual practice in essence. It's an act of devotion because you are filling your finite amount of time in this body with mindsets, actions and activities that nourish you rather than deplete you. When I begin the process of forming a new habit, I choose to approach it as though it is something sacred. A new way of Being that I am calling in and magnetizing into my life. I am attracting it.

In the moment of *making a clear decision to change a habit and devote yourself to that change*, your Being radiates out attraction to that place in time in the future. The sacred act of devotion to the habit change is resetting your inner compass to a new north, and allowing life to then guide you in that direction.

63

One day, you'll wake up and realize that you are where you dreamed of being not so long ago. This is the magic of knowing where you want to go and then always moving forward in that direction; you'll eventually end up where you want to be.

2.   Your family has a lot to do with your habits and the ways in which you live in your body.

The field of epigenetics is quick gaining momentum and shaking up the way we think about how our body is affected by our family and environment. Epigenetics is finding that the genetic expression of every cell in our body is influenced by our environment, and that different genes will be turned 'on' or 'off' depending on their surroundings. The environment you grow up in can make you more or less susceptible to various diseases and ailments. Cancers, diabetes, anxiety, depression, and addictions can all be pointed to epigenetic influences.

One can take this idea one step further and look at how the lived experiences of your parents, grandparents, great-grandparents (and so on) also affect your life. For example, the egg that would become 'You' was in your mother's ovary when she was still in utero in your Grandmother's body. It can be posited that the lived experience of your Grandmother not only had an effect on your Mother's body while she was in utero, but on yours as well when you were an egg. It's important to take into consideration the lives and experiences of your direct family members which may have shaped the way *you* live your life.

The habits of our family members are the easiest for us to fall in line with; and as such, we tend to mimic the lifestyles of our family. We are basically born into a programmed lifestyle and belief-set, and this is not our fault. When we grow into adulthood and move away from our family system, we have the opportunity to recognize the habitual programming that has been played out in our lives and we can choose to make a change.

There are certain struggles one must be aware of as we are making these changes; one of them being the idea of bioelectric entrainment. We know through physics that the human body has a bioelectric field. It can be said that our electric field has a certain frequency or resonance. As we grow up in our family system, our frequency or resonance is entrained with that of our other family members. When we move out on our own and experience other bioelectric frequencies, we begin to notice which ones feel good for us to be in. We can then begin to make changes to recalibrate our bioelectric frequency to match those around us.

At the beginning of this change, the new bioelectric frequency is not very stable, meaning our new habits haven't been well integrated and we are prone to relapse into the old pattern. This is why, with people who begin on a healing, spiritual, or healthy-living path, as soon as they spend time with old friends and family members, their old habits reemerge. What is happening is that the new frequency of the bioelectric field is not strong enough in the body yet to stand alone, and goes back to the way in which it was before. This is the truth behind the phrase, 'old habits die hard'.

I am sharing all of this not to scare you, or tell you not to be around friends from the past or your family as you are making a change. I offer these words, rather, to invite you to be aware of the influence of family systems and bioelectric field resonances as you try to produce change. While you are in the process of reorienting your life to one that supports the health of your body and cervix, you may need to assert boundaries or take more personal space than usual. This is okay. You are forging new habits and recalibrating your bioelectric frequency. You are healing. It is more than okay to take the space you need to do this for yourself.

Behavior Change is Cyclical, Not Linear

Changing habits and behavior can be difficult, especially when it comes to our body, health and even more so, to our sexual nature. Habits and behaviors are like pathways furrowed in our brains, and once a pathway is deeply carved in, it can be (or feel) nearly impossible to forge a new one. While it may feel *impossible*, it *is* definitely possible.

Changing your behavior is a process, and very often we seemingly end up where we began. Many people get frustrated and give up when this happens, but appearing to end up back where you started is actually a part of the process of changing behavior and forging new pathways.

Changing behavior to form new habits is a cyclical process. The lived-experience is akin to a spiral — a three-dimensional spiral — where each time you loop around and end up back where you started, you are in fact *not* where you started, but slightly ahead of where you began. Each time you cycle back to end up back where you began, you are in fact not the same anymore. You've gained experience, knowledge, and wisdom about yourself and how you are in the new habit. You've learned lessons. This is exciting because this means you can employ these new-found insights and wisdom-nuggets in your next attempt.

A model exists to describe the cyclical process of moving through behavior change that I find helpful and want to briefly share with you here. It is called the 'Transtheoretical Model of Behavior Change', but for simplicity's sake we can just call it the 'Model of Behavior Change'. This model, designed and tested through thirty-five years of scientific research, has conceptualized the process of intentional behavior change.[10]

Stages of change are the root of this model. Studies have found that people move through a series of stages when changing their behavior, and these stages are what I want to share with you here, in relation to the healing journey. While the time spent in each stage varies depending on the individual, the tasks required to move through them do not.

The stages of change are as follows: [11]

- Precontemplation (not yet ready): People in this stage do not intend to take any action in the foreseeable future (within the next six months). Being uninformed, or under-informed, about the consequences of behavior or repeated unsuccessful attempts at change may cause a person to exist in this stage.
- Contemplation (getting ready): In this stage, people intend to change in the next six months. They are more aware of the pros of changing and are very aware of the cons. The weighing of pros and cons can lead to doubt and hesitancy, which can then cause people to remain in this stage for a long time. This stage is also defined as chronic contemplation, or procrastination.
- Preparation (ready): Preparation is when people intend to take action in the immediate future (within the next month). Commonly, people have already taken some sort of significant actions in the past year. There is a plan of action such as joining a gym or hiring a coaching and they are ready to initiate it.
- Action: This is the stage where people have made specific changes in their lifestyle within the past six months. These actions must be sufficient in change to reduce risk of disease, etc.; not just small tiny actions that make no difference in the health situation.
- Maintenance: Maintenance is the stage when specific overt modifications in lifestyle have been made and one is working to prevent relapse. In this stage, people are less tempted to relapse and grow more confident that they can carry on their changes.

It is very common (and assumed) that you will cycle through these five stages when making any sort of change in your lifestyle. This is especially true when it comes to changing your lifestyle in regard to your sexual and reproductive health.

Your behaviors, thoughts, mindsets, and personal actions have led you to acquire the diagnosis of HPV and cervical dysplasia (or any other cervical/reproductive condition), and this condition can be reversed through the same means. As you begin to implement the various Cervical Wellness self-care and healing practices, keep in mind these stages of change.

Take a moment and notice where you are in the cycle, yourself. Are you in preparation (reading this book, gathering your tools)? Or are you in contemplation (you are planning and preparing yourself through reading this book and planning on when/where you will get the tools and make changes)? Perhaps you are already in action (taking supplements, changing your diet) but then you fall back into preparation (gathering more tools, learning more information). All of this is okay and to be expected.

Know that you'll fall back and cycle through these stages. Know that you have all the power within you to pick yourself back up and start again. This is the process of healing. Doing it again and again; persevering even when you feel like you want to give up, or when you end up where you perceptually began. Keep going. Keep trying. Keep doing. You will eventually get to where you want to go, and you *will* heal. Just keep going.

You've got this.

PART TWO | ENERGETICS
WHAT LIES BENEATH THE SURFACE

CHAPTER THREE

ENERGETICS OF HPV AND CERVICAL
DYSPLASIA

ENERGY is the underpinning of everything around us. We are all made of trillions of vibrating cells. The choices we make, our behaviors, and the ways in which we think and act each affect our energy. The quality of our energy ultimately leads us in the direction of health or disease. While this book is focused on the physical body and practical application of lifestyle improvements, I feel it's important to address the energetic aspects of HPV and cervical dysplasia. The piece about energetics tends to be the most poignant for most of my clients.

The manifestation of a disease or condition in the physical body is akin to the tip of an iceberg. Underneath the water line is the whole body of the iceberg which constitutes the emotions, beliefs and mindsets tied to the physical manifestation of the disease. The energetics of a situation is the bulk of the problem and once learned about and amended, healing easily follows.

I invite you to think about your body as a castle, and to visualize the round turrets that are usually found on the corners of castles. On these turrets stand sentries — the ones who look out across the land and defend the castle from foreign invaders. These sentries are your immune system. Your immune system is your guardian; the protector of your castle (your body). Your immune system searches and destroys anything resembling an intruder.

The immune system is your boundary system. It differentiates between 'You' and 'other'. If an 'other' (virus, bacteria, pathogen) enters into your body, the immune system notices, activates, attacks and destroys the attacker. This action of our immune system happens on a daily basis. We're continuously exposed to pathogens and our immune system is continuously doing its job in protecting your body (your castle) from being overtaken. The HPV virus is no different than any other pathogen that enters into the body and the immune system does nothing unique or different to ward it off. If this is true, then the questions that remain are:

· What is happening?
· Why are so many women experiencing HPV and being so affected?
· Why now?

Throughout the duration of this next section, I invite you to keep in your mind that the immune system is the guardian system; the boundary between 'You' and 'other', keeping out foreign invaders, and maintaining a healthy balance within the body. Now, let's look at this from an energetic viewpoint.

HPV

When HPV takes over our body and we receive a diagnosis of HPV after a pap test, this is an indication that our 'guardian system' (the immune system) has been let down and our 'guard' has been dropped. Energetically, this is an indication that we have allowed the walls and boundaries of our inner world to be breached and 'invaders' have been allowed to overtake our bodies.

To say it more bluntly: Our boundaries have been crossed. We've either allowed our boundaries to be crossed or our boundaries have been crossed against our will. Given that HPV is a sexually transmitted infection, these boundaries which have been crossed tend to have to do with sexual experiencing.

A question I want to pose for you and invite you to mull over is:

When in the past have you let your guard down with a sexual partner(s) when you weren't 100% ready to?

We can be ready to let our guard down to allow another to enter in. We can lower our boundaries for the sake of intimacy and connection, and consciously welcome another into us [energetically]. Yet very often our boundaries can be crossed when we don't want them to be or are not ready.

When HPV is prevalent in a female body, this is a direct indication to me that there has been a crossing of the boundaries in sexual experiences of the past. The walls of the inner world (our castle) have been broken through and invaded. The energy of that experience created the space for HPV to find a way in to propagate throughout our body.

When our boundaries have been crossed with or without our awareness, this sends a message to our immune system that it doesn't have to work so hard to be the protector anymore. Our immune system takes a cue from our behaviors. If we allow our boundaries to be crossed before we are actually ready to have them be so, our immune system responds and lets down its guard.

When we let down our guard and unconsciously create space within our immune system, the virus we may have been exposed to (even years ago) finds an in. A virus can lurk around in our bodies for years at a time, where, when it discovers a breach in our immune system, it then proliferates in our bodies. If you have HPV, this is a sign that your boundaries have been crossed and your guard has been let down.

When I first came to this understanding, it felt like the walls were closing in around me. I realized how many times in my sexual history I had allowed my boundaries to be crossed when I wasn't 100% ready.

How many times had I allowed someone to penetrate me when I wasn't fully aroused? How many times had I allowed someone to touch me when I actually didn't want to be touched? How many times did I find myself drunk at a party where I made out with the guy I really wasn't interested in that was interested in me? How many times had I allowed someone else's energy to dictate my choices and actions? In all these circumstances, my boundaries had been crossed, and this happening over and over again made space for the HPV to nestle in and stay there.

Whether or not you find this too 'woo-woo' or ungrounded, the truth is that it was only when I realized this and became firm in my decision to have strong energetic boundaries (even in my partnership) that the HPV went away. It's like my immune system said to me, "Oh, you want boundaries now? You want a guardian? Well, before, you were pretty lax in the boundaries, but now I see you are ready to have them again. Okay, I'm back and ready to bolster up, strengthen, and play my role to defend you against the HPV virus."

I'm saying this not to place blame or to point fingers at you, calling out your lack of boundaries. As with everything else in this book, this is an invitation to bring awareness to this aspect of your life and to notice if in your sexual history your boundaries have been crossed. This is also an invitation to notice if you were complicit in any of these experiences and to bring them to light.

Cervical Dysplasia

At its most basic essence, cervical dysplasia is a sign of self-rejection.

When we've let our guard down and allowed our boundaries to be crossed through physical and energetic penetration, we subconsciously punish ourselves. When we've had adverse sexual experiences, we tend to punish ourselves as well. We go over and over in our minds, wondering what we have done wrong; what we could have done differently, lamenting over what we wore that night or whether we were being too flirtatious. "I should have said *No*" or "I should have walked away" are common thoughts to have when our boundaries have been crossed. We ruminate and place the blame on ourselves. This rumination and self-blame leads us to punish ourselves in our minds. As we punish ourselves for what happened, we end up rejecting ourselves. This process can be entirely subconscious.

We reject ourselves because we blame ourselves for what happened. We blame our body and decide not to live in and embody 'down there' anymore. In our conscious awareness, our vaginal canal, vulva, cervix and entire pelvic bowl has become a place of shame, grief and guilt. When we entertain these feelings, we reject our body and our body responds thusly. Our body begins to say, "Wait a minute! Why are you rejecting me?" This is when cervical dysplasia arises.

When I was beginning my healing journey, I hated my reproductive system and sexual organs. I was dealing with irregular menses, sexual traumas, HPV and cervical dysplasia, low libido, having had an abortion, and felt like my reproductive and sexual organs were literal hell. I sometimes even wished I was in a male body so I wouldn't have to deal with all of it. I would take my fists and punch myself in the womb when I was frustrated, because that is how much I loathed and rejected myself. I received the diagnosis of cervical dysplasia year after year, and my frustration with my body only grew in response. My self-rejection deepened. At the peak of this self-rejection, the cervical dysplasia worsened and moved up several grades (CIN 1 -> CIN 2 -> Early CIN 3). I felt like I was at war with myself. This, in fact, is exactly what cancer is. Cancer is nothing more than your body's own cells mutating and turning against the self. Cervical dysplasia happens to be the precursor to cervical cancer.

The process of self-harm (via negative thoughts and self-talk) and self-rejection is detrimental to cervical health. The energy of self-rejection, loathing, shame, anger and hatred towards one's own cervix and reproductive system only exacerbates the problem.

The choice to reject oneself takes a lot of energy. It takes a lot of energy to ignore the pain of internally harming yourself, and this is very depleting on our body. Our body's energy reserves are finite. We have a finite amount of internal resources, and if your resources are being allocated to the cultivation of terrible thoughts about yourself, then that life-force energy cannot go to where it needs to go. Disease and conditions are signs that our body is being depleted and is unable to use its internal resources to maintain health and wellness through its natural cycles of growth and regeneration.

These thoughts are embodied through our conscious denial of our pain. Turning a blind eye to the beliefs which are at the center of our pain (which tends to be within the pelvic region of our body) is felt in the body. The body is very intelligent and knows when you are rejecting it. When we reject a portion of our body, our body experiences this rejection and begins to cry out for you to love it, notice it and accept it. This 'crying out for attention' *is* unwellness and disease.

Any sort of disease or condition in the body, particularly in the female reproductive system, is your body crying out for attention. It's your body yearning for you to turn inward to listen to what it is trying to tell you. What is the message your body is trying to share with you?

The cry of your body becomes worse when months (and maybe even years) go by where you are not listening to it. With cervical dysplasia, the cells of the transformation zone begin to become more upset (dysplastic). Your body produces more and more abnormal cells

77

with the hope that you'll finally connect with your cervix and say, 'OK. I am paying attention. What are you trying to tell me?' Cervical cancer is the last hope the body has that you will actually pay attention to it. Cervical cancer emerges when you continue to reject yourself and don't listen.

A Lineage of Self-Rejection

The internal choice and process of self-rejection can be passed down from Mother to daughter. While on my healing journey, I began to think about my Mother and how she talked about and related to her own sexuality and sexual experiences. I thought about what I knew about her boundaries when she was a young woman. I dove deeper into what I had learned about *my* body and sexual organs from my Mother (and what she had learned from hers) and it all became quite clear.

It was easy for me to reject myself because that is what I was taught: To blame myself and subconsciously punish myself for what happened (whatever the experience might be).

Another question I have for you to think about is:

Did your Mother have a healthy relationship with her body and boundaries? Did your Grandmother (Mother's mother)?

The answer to these questions may help to give you clues as to where the habit of self-rejection may have come from.

CHAPTER FOUR

ENERGETICS OF WOMEN'S HEALTH

OUR bodies are miraculous. They regenerate and grow new cells all the time. Our body has the ability to heal itself — as long as we get out of its way. Our bodies can handle a lot more than we give them credit for, and in looking at the energetics of Women's health, we can have a greater understanding of how we can support our body to do what it does naturally, and that is to heal.

We will look at what the energy of Women's health entails, as well as what you can begin to think about and take into consideration as you embark on your healing journey.

Feminine Body Intelligence

Females have the capacity to 'know' or have a 'knowing' with their bodies as well as their minds. This is due to the fact that female brains are set up and wired differently than male brains. The corpus callosum (the part of the brain connecting the two hemispheres) is thicker in females than males, relative to brain size.[20] Some claims have been made stating that this creates more connectivity and available neural pathways between and amongst the two hemispheres of the brain, due to this difference in ratio.[21] Plainly stated, females are more easily able to access information in both hemispheres of the brain at the same time. This supports the notion that male-bodied people tend to be more inclined toward singular-focused activities; whereas, female-bodied people have an easier time multitasking and holding multiple trains of thought at once.

I've personally noticed that Women *do* think and process thoughts differently than males. Females tend to think and process in a cyclical way, accessing both hemispheres at the same time. Emotional and relational experiences are incorporated in the processing and thinking, as well as felt- and lived-experiences of the body. Women tend to combine logical and emotional reasoning in conversations, discussions and decision making. It's also known that we tend to go into more detail and access past stories and experiences when describing something or giving instructions. Men tend to be very succinct and straightforward in their descriptions and directions. They tend not to bring in emotions and feeling-tones to the dialogue.

[I recognize these are blanket statements, and aren't necessarily true for everyone. I include these broad-stroke understandings to provide context for the sake of this book and discussion.]

When thinking about how Women process, communicate and express themselves in the world, we *must* give our bodies credit for the innate wisdom they hold. This wisdom comes in the form of the emotional, relational, and lived experiences which we bring to the forefront of our expression and communication style.

Feminine body intelligence is accessing and allowing these 'illogical' internal experiences to be expressed. We don't have to know *why* our heart is racing, or *why* we feel like crying or feel excited. We're able to *be* in those experiences without having a logical understanding, and only after we've allowed ourselves to *just be* with what we are feeling, *then* the mental understanding arises. Feeling really mad or angry, and just sitting with it — *being with it* — is tapping into this feminine body intelligence.

Feelings are your body's way of communicating to you. Unlike our Mind, which can have a very distinct 'voice' (at least mine does!), our body doesn't have a 'voice' that communicates to us via words or language that is understood with logical reasoning. Our body's voice is the feelings, the emotions and the felt-experience of the body itself.

Feminine body intelligence permits feelings and emotions *to be* without trying to silence them. When we allow them to naturally rise up and we 'listen' to them via sitting quietly, taking a bath, or journaling, we tap into this feminine body intelligence and make ourselves available to receive the messages of our Body.

I've come to understand that, as a person with a female body, I have three different 'brains'. I have my brain 'brain', my heart 'brain', and my womb 'brain'. These three locations in the body are where I can tap into and access intelligence. The brain 'brain' is where I can access analytical thought processes, problem solve, and perform logical tasks such as budgeting or planning a schedule for a project. The heart 'brain' is where I'm able to tap into the feelings of love, connection and relationship. Then there is the womb 'brain'. A past client of mine developed a word I love called 'wombtuition'. The 'womb brain' residing within our pelvic bowl is the ultimate feminine body intelligence access point. The womb is the center of our creative fire, where Women cultivate and gestate a sense of *being* and sense of creation. Male bodies also have the same energetic access point, only it's different in form and nature. When we're able to bring our awareness to our womb and ask, "Womb, what do you know? What are you trying to show me?" The answers that arise tend to be exactly what we need to hear. The intelligence harbored in this place of the body is highly potent.

Thoughts Embodied

There exists a cultural belief that the female body is inherently 'abnormal'. Every single aspect of the female body experience has been pathologized — birth, menstruation, pregnancy, and menopause. These experiences are treated as though they are 'conditions' which need to be dealt with, and consequently our bodies are treated as such. It wasn't too long ago where, when a Woman experienced premenstrual symptoms or anxiety after childbirth, she was deemed 'hysterical' and sent to an insane asylum.[22] As hard as we try, those of us with female bodies internalize the belief that our body is 'wrong'.

We are taught that femalehood is 'dirty'. For example, we are told via marketing that we must work hard to protect the outside world from knowing when we are bleeding. If we spring a 'leak', it's assumed we need to feel mortified. We are conditioned to believe that we must 'smell fresh' and that our natural body odors are unpleasant to the nose of the opposite sex. Deodorized douches and aluminum-laden deodorants are pushed onto us to make us smell like 'rain' or 'fresh spring'. Media tells us we need to appear 'clean' and we are sold dozens of products to remove or change our body hair. These cultural beliefs have led to a population of Women who believe that they are inherently 'imperfect' and must do something to help make themselves 'perfect'.

These cultural beliefs have led to most Women having terrible thoughts about their body. Ingrained beliefs transform into thought processes which run on and on in the background of our mind. These programs lead to a significant amount of internal pain and self-rejection.

We may not even be aware of these thoughts. They may be subconscious. However, when we have the same thought over and over again, and think about it often, it eventually manifests into something physical, such as a condition or ailment. The logical reasoning goes: If beliefs become thoughts and thoughts become something physical, then beliefs manifest into the physical.

Energy-Centers, Health and Disease

*While I am not Indian in heritage, I find that the teachings of the energy centers (chakras) of the body are quite profound and influential. I am in no way claiming to be a teacher of Ayurveda and Indian spiritualism. To find classical and well-trained teachers of these practices, please go to the reference section.

The energy centers in the lower half of our body set the stage for either disease or health in the female reproductive system. These energy centers have been recorded throughout time, most notably in the Hindu tradition of India. These centers or chakras are said to be spinning wheels through which prana (or life force energy) flow. The chakra system is comprised of seven 'centers' found within the human body system. Each chakra corresponds to specific organs, as well as physical, emotional, psychological, and spiritual states of being, and they influence all the areas of your life. This system originated in India and founded an ancient text called the Vedas, written between 1500 and 500 BC.

There isn't any Western scientific 'evidence' that translates spiritual energy into physical manifestation; however, the Western adoption of practices such as yoga and reiki are a testament to Westerners' desire for these sorts of teachings. It is believed and practiced that when the chakras are open and aligned, our energy is free-flowing and allows life-force energy to flow through. When the chakras are blocked, a person may experience a variety of mental, emotional and physical un-wellness, depending on which chakra the energy cannot flow through.

The first three chakras are the ones we will be discussing here. These energy centers are located at the base of the spine, the sacrum and above the naval.

A basic overview of the first three chakras:

The first chakra, also called the Root chakra or Muladhara in Sanskrit, is located at the very base of your spine, near your tailbone.

84

Other body areas that are correlated with this energy center are the rectum, hip joints, blood and immune system. The energy associated with the root chakra has to do with home, our tribe, and sense of safety. Any sort of problems or issues having to do with unresolved family issues and physical survival issues (i.e. one's house, family, sexual identity or race) are represented here.

The second chakra, also called the Sacral Chakra or Svadhisthana, is located right below the belly button and is associated with the pelvic bowl (bladder and appendix) and reproductive organs (vulva, vagina, uterus, cervix, and ovaries). The energy associated with the sacral chakra deals with our outer drives in the world, our identity as a human, and what we do with it. This chakra brings creative energy to help us enjoy life. It is the home of the creative life-force energy that motivates us to enjoy the fruits of our labor and to experience pleasurable activities such as sex. The health of this area is affected by the degree to which our relationships are based on issues of trust, control, blame, and guilt.

The third chakra, also called the Solar Plexus Chakra or Manipura, is located in the center of the belly button and extends up to the breastbone. The areas in the body associated with this energy center include the gallbladder, liver, pancreas, stomach and small intestine. This chakra deals with our self-esteem, self-confidence, self-respect, and personal power.

The quality of the third chakra depends on the quality of the first and second chakras. In order to have high self-esteem, a Woman must feel secure in the world (associated with the root chakra) and must have relationships based upon mutual respect and support (associated with the sacral chakra). These three power centers happen to encapsulate the entirety of the reproductive system. Although the second chakra is the power center of the reproductive system itself, the first and third chakras inform what is happening there. All the unresolved stresses of our early physical life related to people, events, memories, and experiences pull energy from these three lower power centers, ultimately creating disease and un-wellness.

Healing these power centers can only occur in the present, when we allow ourselves to feel, express and release emotions stored there from the past that we have suppressed or tried to forget. When we repeatedly say to ourselves 'No I don't want to look at that. No I don't want to feel that. I'll process that later', we are continuously repressing the experiences that our body wants us to remember and process. You may try your hardest to 'forget' in your mind, but your body will never ever forget. Our body never forgets.

I have a theory as to how disease and un-wellness manifest in the body, coinciding with this idea that the body never forgets. I call this *emotional tethering*.

Healing Yourself from the Past

Emotional tethering is being energetically tethered to the past. Now, I'm going to get a little quantum physic-y here, so just bear with me.

We are in this physical body in the third dimension, and are moving through Time and Space. I invite you to think about this Time/Space continuum as a solid 'loaf', and we are moving *through* the loaf as we live our lives and age (stay with me here). Our body has experiences as we move through Time (time is passing). These experiences can be pleasurable, or can be traumatic and adverse. When we have traumatic or adverse experiences and we don't allow ourselves the opportunity to integrate them into our body, we can become tethered.

86

What happens here is that a piece of *You* (your life-force energy) becomes stuck in that moment in Time, in the Space-Time loaf, whenever the traumatic/adverse experience occurred. As you continue to move forward through Time, that piece of You is still stuck way back in the past. It can be a week ago, a year ago, or even twenty years ago, but that piece of You is still way back there, while the rest of you is moving forward. You become energetically tethered to that moment in Time, and the longer that tether gets, the more it strains the physical body. The more strain there is on the body, the more your body calls out to you to look at it where the tether is still attached, so that you can unhook from that moment in Time and bring that piece of you back.

While I was healing my cervix, I looked way back to when I was four or five years old and I was shamed by a friend's Mother for exploring sexuality and sensuality with that friend. This experience was so traumatic for me that from that moment on, I felt shameful of arousal and my sexual organs. I had an extremely difficult time connecting to my vulva well into adulthood, and lamented at being in a female body because of this. I figured out that a piece of me was still stuck at the age of four when I was shamed by my friend's Mother. I realized that no matter how many times I had remembered that memory, I hadn't ever actually processed it. So I had to do the work to remember, to cry, to release, to express these feelings of shame towards my body and sexuality, all of which I never had the opportunity to do when the experience had originally occurred.

While in the middle of this processing, I literally felt the 'hook' in the past 'unhook', the energy return to me, and lo and behold I felt better. The ways in which I associated with my sexuality and sexual nature shifted almost immediately, and my body was able to allocate that strained life-force energy elsewhere.

So, what do you need to untether yourself from?

The first question I ask is:

Where and what in the past do you need to look at to unhook your energy from, so that that piece of you, that life-force energy (your vital inner resources), can return to your body? (When this energy is returned to your Body, it can then do what it needs to do in order to return balance and healing to your physical body-system in current time.)

Some tools you can use to untether yourself from the past and return energy to your reproductive system include:

Experiential Processing

Make a list of every single sexual experience you have ever had, starting from early childhood. Write down when you started to masturbate, when you started becoming aware of feeling 'turned on' and aroused, when the first time was where someone who wasn't you had touched your body (though perhaps not when your parents helped you as an infant/child), when you lost your virginity, and what your sexual experiences were as a teenager and early adult. Actively remember everything and write it down. Make a timeline, a list, or any other way to organize your experiences. Take a look at the list and notice, where are the charges?

When you come to a memory that you cringe around or want to 'skip over' and not write down, there may be a tether there. The process of actively remembering and, essentially, reliving those experiences in an intentional way, will help your body to integrate and bring back those tethers. Touch and massage your body as these charges emerge. It is important that we address them on a somatic level. Stop and do some yoga, dance or other conscious movement.

Some of these tethers can be super strong and thick; whereas others may be fine, baby-hair tethers. Yet, each and every tether drains the energy of our reproductive system, so bringing them all back is your responsibility.

Using Crystals inside the Vaginal Canal

Each type of crystal has different healing properties:

Jade: Considered the health, wealth and longevity stone and to have a steady, gentle pulse of healing energy. Carries the energy of the Earth, which nurtures, soothes, and uplifts the heart.

Rose Quartz: Opens the heart to all types of love. Helps to raise self-esteem, restore confidence, and balance emotions.

Obsidian: A powerful grounding stone, it connects you to your root. Aids in protection and the clearing of dense, psychic smog from your aura (attachments, disharmony, old patterns, negative emotions, and anything else you're hiding away).

*Note: Jade is typically used intravaginally; however, one can begin with rose quartz. Obsidian is an advanced stone to use intravaginally and is recommended for use only after having used jade for some time. Also, do NOT purchase 'cheap' stones. There are a plethora of fake yoni-eggs made from other types of stones or even plastic. It's highly important that you make sure the source of your stone has a high-vibration and is of certified quality. See the resource section for my recommended sources.

What I love about using crystals shaped as eggs intra-vaginally is not only how they assist in bringing awareness down to your pelvic region, but also the poetic beauty of their shape. They support us in unlocking the stories that are harbored there, needing to be witnessed.

If you are feeling ready to move on from the egg, a crystal wand (dildo) is a wonderful tool to use with intra-vaginal and cervical acupressure. Gently pressing the tip of the wand in different areas of your vaginal canal (with loving awareness) is a method of use in unlocking the tension and memories stored within the body, and thus going a little deeper than the eggs can. Intentional physical intra-vaginal massage can bring forth what needs to be healed.

Go slowly, and be gentle (especially on the cervix).

Writing Letters

Write a letter to another person whom you feel may have harmed you, or to yourself for not having listened to the voice of your body in the past. These letters do not need to be sent to or seen by anyone but you. However, sending a letter speaking your truth to someone who may have [knowingly or unknowingly] harmed you in the past is extremely empowering if you feel so inclined.

This sense of empowerment is especially palpable when you write a letter to someone who has sexually assaulted, harassed or harmed you in some way. Your body may still be experiencing the fear and pain of the past event; especially if you have never expressed your feelings to this person before. Writing a letter and getting it out into words what happened, how it affected you, and your true feelings on the matter will help you to release the emotional tethers to the past as well as to any associated individuals. This, then, allows your own sense of inner power to return.

*Note: Only send the letter if you feel like that is right for you and your process. Even just writing the letter and not sending it is powerful.

Keep Track of Your Dreams

As you are in the process of untethering yourself from the past, you may begin to process this energy in your subconscious. Indication of this happening will appear during your dreamtime. Pay special attention to the items and locations in your dreams, as well as any people that may show up. Keep a dream journal. Write them down as soon as you wake up. You can look back over your dreams to notice any patterns or manifestations on a physical level.

You may also begin to dream of a person who has harmed you in the past or whom who you have tethers to. They may still be drawing energy from you through the tether, and as you work on releasing yourself, they may subconsciously reach out and try to stop you from cutting them off. Keep going. This means it's working.

Practice Saying Your No

Learn what 'NO' feels like in your body. Here is a short exercise you can do to learn what 'NO' actually *feels* like.

Stand straight up but relaxed, with your eyes closed.

Ask your Body, "Body, show me what yes feels like." Wait to receive a response.

Ask your Body, "Body, show me what no feels like." Wait to receive a response.

Ask your Body, "Body, show me what neutral feels like." Wait to receive a response.

This process will help you to differentiate between these three states. This way, when you come across a circumstance where your body is clearly telling you 'NO', you will understand what it is saying and will then be able to voice it aloud.

I once heard a saying that I now love, that goes, "If it's not a *hell yes*, then it's a *no*." Listen for that 'hell yes'.

Acceptance and Forgiveness

Forgiveness is not for the other person. It is for you. By forgiving and releasing your heart from any negative feelings which may be draining you of vital life force energy, you will *free yourself* from the past. This is ultimately what untethering is: Looking into the past to

91

see/remember what happened, accepting that it happened, and forgiving *yourself* for what transpired. Forgiveness is unburdening yourself from the mental process of repeating the experience over and over again in your mind.

A journal question: *What is one thing that, if you fully accept and forgive, will free you?*

PART THREE |
CERVICAL SELF-CARE

I INVITE...

...all those with cervixes to engage in the Cervical Wellness Self-Care Method. These are lifestyle practices to take into consideration for your cervical health.

The cervix and cervical health are intricately linked with overall immunological health. Much of what I'll be talking about from here on out has to do with supporting your immune system so that it can naturally fight off HPV.

For those of you who have cervical dysplasia and yet have been told that you don't have HPV or are currently not expressing HPV at the moment, this is still for you. What could have happened is that you've had HPV in the past and as such, have led the transformation zone of your cervix to become compromised. Even if you've already suppressed HPV and it is not showing up as being 'active' in your pap-tests, these lifestyle practices are still for you.

I'm going to repeat myself here and say once again that cervical health is intricately linked to immune health. What I share with you encompasses both of these body systems: reproductive health and immune health.

This information comprises all of what I personally did to heal myself. Everything I'm listing, here in this section, is what I used to heal seven years of HPV and cervical dysplasia. Now, this is not to say that there isn't more that can be done. I have included other tools and resources in the Self-Care and Ritual Toolkit in the back of this book; however, this is what I teach and what I know works.

CHAPTER FIVE

PRELIMINARY STEPS:

GETTING TO KNOW YOUR CERVIX

Touching Your Cervix

I highly encourage and advocate for you to spend some time getting
to know your cervix yourself, before you even begin to think about
going down the route of Western medical treatment. Getting to know
your cervix in an intimate and heart-centered way will begin the process
of *actually healing*.

I invite all Women to take the time to touch their own cervix
for the purpose of connection and exploration. Touching and gently
massaging your cervix with your own fingers will initiate a process of
inner-world connection that we, as Women, were never given
permission to do.

Touching your own cervix with your own hand is one of the
most healing things we can do. Our cervix tends to only be touched by
others. Think about it. How many people have touched your cervix?
Doctors? Lovers? How many people have already felt inside your inner
world when you yourself perhaps have not?

Our cervix is calling out for us to connect to her, get to know
her, and to establish a relationship with her. A way to do this is to touch
her. Have you ever put your fingers inside your own vaginal canal
without the intention of receiving pleasure or checking your cervical
fluid for fertility awareness? Have you ever put your fingers inside just
for the sake of feeling what is going on in there and connecting to this
place in your body that is perceived as dark and hidden?

This is the first step in all Cervical Self Care: getting to know
your inner world in a loving and friendly way. For many Women, this is

the scariest part of cervical self-care. This is why I invite you to do it —
to overcome the fear of connecting to the Cervix for yourself.

Invitation: Find time one evening to get to know your cervix in an
intimate way. You will learn what it is like to have your cervix touched
by yourself, by practicing cervical self-exploration. It is time to develop
a loving relationship with her. Set up a nice space, light a candle, burn
some sage, and prepare for a most sacred introduction.

11 Steps for Cervical Self-Exploration

1. Wash your hands
2. Set up a nice ambiance — you are meeting her for the first time
   (candles, music, being alone)
3. You can squat OR lay on your back, knees splayed, pillows
   supporting your knees and lower back
4. Talk with your body, and let her know what you are about to
   do. Spend some time and ask your body for permission to enter
5. Blow some kisses on your hands
6. Gently insert 1-2 fingers in your vagina, and move them up until
   you reach a stopping point: THAT'S YOUR CERVIX!
7. Gently explore what she feels like
8. Can you feel the Os? Is she open or closed? Is there fluid or
   does she feel dry? (these tell you the state of your fertility)
9. How is your body responding to the touch? Are there emotions
   arising? Is there fear? Breathe. Be with it. This is an important
   introduction.
10. When you feel complete, thank your cervix for her participation.
    Remove your fingers, and wash your hands
11. Give thanks for this new connection.

Ask for a Mirror at Your Next Gynecological Appointment

Lack of knowledge regarding the cervix is an epidemic among Women. For decades, Women of all ages, races, and ethnicities have gone to the doctor for their routine yearly pap-test, with little to no understanding as to what is being checked or why. It has become a 'given' in our society that Women need to have this exam, and no one takes the time to explain to us what exactly is going on.

One way to remedy the lack of awareness we have about our cervix is to ask for a mirror the next time you get a pap or pelvic exam done. Each exam room is equipped with a hand-mirror which you can ask to use to see your cervix the next time you find yourself open with a speculum. This simple request will deepen your connection to your body and cervix, and support you in establishing a loving relationship with your pelvic bowl. You will get to see your other Face.

The top three reasons why I invite you to ask for a mirror:

1. *It helps to heal our relationship to our bodies*

The truth is that when we are able to gaze up and witness with our *very own eyes* a place in our body that is shrouded in fear, shame, regret, and guilt, we are able to initiate the process of healing our relationship to it. Healing our relationship to our body is the #1 task we as modern Women have in front of us during this time in history. By gathering up the courage to look with our own eyes at the place in our body we've been taught to fear will dissipate the veil of darkness which has been placed over ourselves, and bring to new light who we are and what our Body — our very own Body — looks like.

2. It puts you in charge of how the pap goes

Western medical doctors are busy. On average, MDs and Nurse practitioners have roughly eight to ten minutes to give to each patient, and this small allotment of time leads to gynecological exams feeling rushed, forced, and sometimes even intrusive. There is no time for Women to prepare for the invasiveness of being penetrated, let alone having their cervix scraped and swabbed.

Asking for a mirror puts you in the driver's seat of what's happening. When you request a mirror and the doctor or nurse practitioner hands it to you, you are then the one who dictates for how long you choose to look. The doctors cannot rip the mirror out of your hands or tell you to stop.

When that mirror is handed to you, take your time. Take a breath. Prepare for a sacred introduction. You are going to witness your inner world for the very first time. This is a special moment. It's like seeing a newborn baby for the first time, or a long-lost family member — except this time, it is YOU.

When you do put the mirror down there to take a look, take your time. I invite you to really gaze at your cervix. Take in the details; imprint them in your memory. This is a special moment for you and your body. Don't be afraid to relish in it.

Your practitioner may ask you to hurry along, and get fidgety. They may seem annoyed that you asked for the mirror, for this will take up their precious time. Pay them no mind. This is *your* experience, *your* body, and *your* sacred introduction. The practitioner will be fine. Remember, they are there to serve *you*, and *not* the other way around.

3. It helps to make your reproductive system and the pap a little less scary

No one really *enjoys* pap-tests. They are invasive, intrusive, and sometimes even traumatic. Yet when you gaze at your cervix in the mirror, you'll see that your body is actually really beautiful. You'll see that your cervix is a small little pink mound that is moist with a hole in the middle.

If you have cervical dysplasia, you may see the dysplastic cells as white spots on your cervix, or display as a darker pink area around the os — but this is okay! In fact, seeing the truth of your situation can be a healing experience. Imagine a child who has skinned their knee. Besides a bandage, sometimes the child just wants you (the adult) to look at the 'boo-boo' and tell them it will be okay. Your cervix is no different.

When you gaze upon your cervix, you will see how it is not the 'big bad wolf' living in there, but rather a small, gentle yet powerful, sacred portal, and not just any sacred portal, but *your* sacred portal.

The experience of witnessing your cervix yourself will help you to feel more empowered in your body, putting you in the driver's seat of the exam experience, and bringing a greater sense of peace and ease to the general fear of the situation. If you don't have the opportunity to gaze upon your cervix for several months, do not worry. This is a standing invitation and one that you can engage in at any point throughout your Cervical Wellness journey.

I do want to note that there are such things as 'cervical self-exam kits'. These kits include a speculum, mirror and flashlight so that you can look at and gaze upon your cervix yourself in the comfort of your own home. You can find more information about cervical self-exam kits in the 'Resources' section of this book.

CHAPTER SIX

LIFESTYLE PRACTICES FOR CERVICAL SELF-CARE

I am a firm believer in our body's natural ability to heal itself. Through our lifestyle, we can allow our body to do what it does naturally, and that is to heal and regenerate.

Nutritional Choices

THE first step in any type of health and wellness lifestyle change is with nutritional choices. There are many different ideas as to what foods are best for the body, and many different diets people choose to ascribe to for health and wellness purposes.

In Cervical Wellness, I invite people to choose foods that *boost* the immune system, which in turn support cervical health.

I recommend transitioning to a healthy, nourishing diet of organic wholefoods such as vegetables, fruits, nuts, saturated fats and proteins. Eating foods which support the immune system and reduce inflammation (the nemesis of the immune system) will help the cervix to regenerate healthy cells in the transformation zone.

I also recommend eliminating foods in the diet which promote inflammation, such as cane sugar, GMO corn and wheat, deep fried foods, and dairy. Eliminating all food that increase the likelihood of inflammation supports the body's ability to keep its immune system functioning properly, as well as nourish the cervix.

When thinking about what to eat to support cervical wellness, choose foods high in:

Ø *Beta-carotene*: yellow-orange vegetables or fruits like carrots, cantaloupe, peaches, squash

Ø *Folic acid*: dark leafy vegetables (kale, cabbage, broccoli, cauliflower, Swiss chard) and asparagus

Ø *Vitamin C*: citrus fruits

Ø *Lycopene*: cooked tomato products, rosehips, watermelon, pink grapefruit

Ø *Saturated Fats*: olive oil, coconut oil, avocado oil, ghee, grass fed butter, lard

> o Saturated fats support your cellular structure. Each cell is encased in a lipid-layer, which is saturated fat. Each of your nerves is lined and encased in saturated fat as well, via the myelin sheath. Saturated fat is for whole-body health.

Ø *Calcium*: Whole milk-dairies, beans, almonds, bok choy, and dark leafy greens, such as spinach and kale

Ø *Antioxidants*: Fruits such as berries, cherries, tomatoes; and vegetables, such as squash and bell pepper. Raw cacao is another amazing source of antioxidants.

You also want to:

Ø Eat lean meats, cold-water fish (salmon, cod, sardines), or beans for protein. Choose animal products only from reputable, sustainable, and conscious sources (no torture-meat please). Grass-fed, pastured and wild are ideal.

Ø Avoid refined foods, such as white breads, pastas, and sugar, and reduce or eliminate trans-fatty acids found in commercially baked goods, such as cookies, crackers, cakes, French fries, onion rings, donuts, processed foods, and margarine. Sugar and refined foods create inflammation in the body and pull vital internal resources away from your immune system and cervix.

Ø Avoid alcohol (especially beer and liquor). I don't advocate for you to be a teetotaler, but do be aware as to how much alcohol you consume. Alcohol greatly impacts immune health and causes inflammation throughout the body system.

You can find some sample recipes which are beneficial for cervical health in the Self-Care and Ritual Toolkit.

Drink Clean Water… and Lots of it!

I recently learned how it is posited that 85% of Americans are chronically dehydrated. While I don't know the source of this statistic, it sure does ring true. We simply do not drink enough water throughout our days.

Most people begin their days with a cup of coffee or tea, without realizing that their body has just undergone 6+ hours without water (while they slept) and that they've awoken dehydrated.

Our bodies *must* have water in order to function properly and regenerate. The human body is made up of roughly 55-70% water. If we do not have enough water in our system, our body becomes taxed and is not able to function in the way that it should. Without water, our body system is unable to be lubricated and do what it needs to do, like regenerate new, healthy cells in the cervix. The importance of drinking enough water cannot be expressed enough.

Even more so, we need to be drinking water with minerals in it. Minerals in water actually help your kidneys up-take the water and keep you hydrated. When you drink water without minerals in it, it will quickly pass through your system and you'll urinate it out. For many of us, we're drinking the necessary water, but our body isn't absorbing it like it should as the water we're drinking lacks the essential minerals for absorption.

Also, most of the water found in taps has been processed and chemically 'purified'. Many cities put fluoride in their water (a neurotoxin which accumulates in the pineal gland in the brain and calcifies it) as well as other chemicals like chlorine. This isn't the water you want.

Ideally, you'll drink natural spring water which is sourced straight from the Earth and contains all of the natural minerals and constituents. However, I understand this may not be available for everyone.

One way to counteract this perpetual dehydration via lack of minerals is to drink a glass of water upon waking with a pinch of sea salt in it. Sea salt (Himalayan pink salt, Celtic sea salt) puts minerals into the water to help your body absorb it. All you need is a small pinch. Any more than that and the water may taste salty.

Another thing to take into consideration is to not drink *ice cold water*. Ice cold water shocks the digestive system. Since a large portion of your immune health is centered in the gut, it is important not to make this place in your body work harder than it has to. Drinking room-temperature, warm or even hot water is best for the body-system.

My morning routine consists of waking up, turning on the water kettle, and pouring myself a 16 oz glass of warm/hot water that I then put a pinch of salt in. Sometimes I add a ½ teaspoon of apple cider vinegar (for probiotics) or a drop of iodine (for thyroid health), but baseline I drink warm salted water. I do this every day before I even THINK about putting anything else in my body, especially caffeine.

Reduce Your Stress

Stress is a major cause of immune-function suppression. When you're stressed out and anxious, your body is thrown into a sympathetic nervous response — or 'fight, flight or freeze'. This state of being causes your body to create hormones that are taxing and exhausting. This response is supposed to occur only when there is a 'threat', yet in today's wild and crazy world, we find ourselves constantly in this fight or flight response.

A 2008 study found that heightened levels of perceived stress are associated with an impaired HPV-specific immune response for women with cervical dysplasia.[15] When women experience stress, their bodies are unable to fight off the viral infection of HPV which eventually leads to cervical dysplasia. Overall immune-system health is imperative in staving off HPV and cervical abnormalities.

Cervical healing occurs when the parasympathetic response (think 'rest and digest') is triggered in the nervous system. This is when the body is relaxed and able to process and repair itself. It's imperative to find ways to relax and feel good in your body. Develop a self-care practice that feels nourishing to your heart and body.

Meditate. Explore yoga, breath work, or martial arts. Go for hikes, take baths, perform self-massage with herbal body-oil or go and get a massage. Make tea and chat with a friend. Do whatever makes you feel good and loved, and do it often. When you reconnect to what brings you a sense of love and joy, you flood your body with hormones like serotonin, dopamine, and oxytocin which make you feel happy, connected and loved. This will, in turn, help your body relax, giving it the much-needed time and space to self-heal from the HPV virus. Turn on that parasympathetic nervous response and support your immune system to perform its service.

I tell all my clients that engaging in stress-reducing activities is non-negotiable. It's important to make stress reduction a top priority. You can be doing all the steps, taking the herbs, doing the practices and connecting to your cervix, yet if you are stressed out, it will not matter.

Stress reduction is the basis of all cervical self-care. It's important you treat it as medicine, just like you would any other medication.

Some activities I recommend to reduce stress include the following:

Ø Acupuncture

Ø Hot bath with Epsom/sea salt

Ø Soaking in mineral springs/swimming in wild water

Ø Walk in the forest, near a body of water, or anywhere in nature

Ø Sleeping

Ø Listening to binaural tones/calming music

Ø Sauna/steam room

Ø Massage

Herbal Medicine

There is little doubt that plants were the first sources of medicine. Even animals have been observed to use them intuitively to treat severe wounds and maladies, and for more than simple nourishment. Herbal medicine is one of the oldest forms of medicine practiced by humans in all of history. Hieroglyphs, drawings, and inscriptions of various plants in medicinal form have been found in ancient sites around the world. This form of healing stretches back across time and connects us to our more primitive ways. The history of herbal medicine dates back to the very beginning of humanity.

Mother Earth knows how to support us. Our planet does this by providing beautiful plants which help us heal and regenerate in a healthy way. In herbalism, there is an understanding that the health and wellness of a single individual has an effect on the wellbeing of the community, and places attention on finding and treating the root cause of a problem. Herbs are most effective on the physical level of a human, yet there is a deeply-rooted spiritual aspect to herbal medicine as well. Many indigenous traditions consider herbal medicine 'plant-spirit medicine' and that by working with and ingesting parts of different plants, one would consume the quality of their 'spirit'.

Above all, herbal medicine is the medicine of nature. It is based upon the characteristics and archetypal essences of all matter on Earth. In most herbal medicine practices around the world, all organ systems of the body are associated and interact with the four seasons and elements of our planet (Earth, Air, Fire, Water, Metal, Wood). Other factors taken into consideration include various tastes and temperatures our body senses experience, temperaments and tendencies (rising, floating, condensing, sinking) and the concepts of movement/stagnation. [12] These practices take into consideration the cyclical aspects of nature and the predictable sequences that nature follows. If it's done in nature, then it's done in our body.

Herbs are another name for parts of plants that have been used in healing remedies. An herb can be any of the following:

An angiosperm (i.e., a flowering plant), shrub, tree, moss, lichen, fern, algae, seaweed, or fungus. The herbalist may use the entire plant or just the flower, fruits, leaves, twigs, bark, roots, rhizomes, seeds, or exudates (e.g. tapped and purified maple syrup), or a combination of parts. [13]

These parts may be used fresh, dried, or powdered. Herbs can be applied topically or can be taken internally to treat a wide range of physical, emotional, mental and spiritual symptoms. Whole or chopped herbs can be used in infusions (steeped as tea) or decoctions (simmered over low heat). Herbs can also be processed into tinctures, oils, oil infusions, and salves to then be turned into various wellness products for the body.

The following herbs have been shown to be beneficial for cervical, reproductive and immunological health. Alongside each name is a description of each herb's beneficial properties, as well as recommended ways to use them.

Goldenseal: Goldenseal is supportive of mucous membranes and in treating microbial and viral infections. Use goldenseal powders in a douche, or drink goldenseal root tea. Please note, this plant is considered endangered, so please purchase from a reputable source.

Calendula: Calendula is anti-inflammatory and antiviral, making it a great ally in healing HPV and cervical dysplasia. Use calendula in a vaginal steam or drink as a tea or tincture.

Nettle: Nettle root (not the leaves) supports Women's hormonal health by decreasing the levels of estrogen metabolites in the body. Use nettle root in a tea or tincture.

Raspberry Leaf: Raspberry leaf tightens and tones the uterine and pelvic muscles, supports fertility and is high in iron. Use raspberry leaf as an infusion and drink as a tea.

Ginseng: Ginseng supports proper immune function, elevates mood, cleanses the blood, balances hormones and fights off infections. Use ginseng as a tea, tincture or supplement.

Lavender: Lavender helps relax the body which can support overall immune health. Lavender can relieve pain, improves brain function, treats anxiety and is overall beneficial for Women's health. Use as an essential oil, or in a vaginal steam.

Rose: Rose boosts the immune system, alleviates inflammation, reduces stress (also supporting immune functioning) and is rich in powerful antioxidants called 'catechin polyphenols' which have been proven to prevent cancer. Use rose in a tea infusion, or in a vaginal steam.

Marigold: Marigold is anti-inflammatory, and supports wound healing. Use as an infusion tea, douche or vaginal steam.

Pau d'Arco: Pau d'Arco has been shown to fight cancer and inflammation. It provides antiviral and antifungal properties, and detoxifies the body. Make an infusion and drink as a tea or use in a douche.

Oregano: Oregano has been shown to be antimicrobial, antioxidant, and relieves menstrual cramp pain. Use as a body oil or in an infusion.

Rosemary: Rosemary reduces stress, balances hormones, boosts our immunity and is antimicrobial. Can be used in foods, body oil, or yoni steam.

Infusions (Teas):

Herbal infusions bring the healing qualities of plants to your whole body-system. Drinking the infusion allows the beneficial qualities of the plants to enter into your circulatory system through the GI-tract, and enhances whole-body wellness. This method is a less direct way to support the cervix, but is beneficial, nonetheless.

The following herbs are examples that can be steeped:

Ø Nettle

Ø Raspberry leaf

Ø Ginseng

Ø Calendula

Ø Lavender

Ø Rose

How to make an infusion:

1. Rinse and awaken herbs in warm water for 10 seconds.
2. Steep herbs in hot (not boiling) water for 3-5 minutes (this is for leaves, and flowers). When using bark or roots, put plant parts in a pot with water. Bring water to a boil and reduce heat to simmer for 15-20 minutes.
3. Strain out herbs.

Drink while hot, and by itself. Do not drink medicinal tea with a meal. When you are drinking tea, just drink the tea. It's medicine.

Vaginal Steams:

Vaginal steams offer a more direct way for the beneficial essential oils of plants to support the cervix. The hot water vapor of steam transfers the essential oils gently into the vagina and onto the cervix.

113

*Do not vaginal steam if you have an IUD, are pregnant, or are menstruating

Vaginal steam herb examples:

Ø Calendula

Ø Lavender

Ø Nettle

Ø Rose

Ø Rosemary

How to Vaginal Steam:

1. Bring a pot of water to a boil. Let cool for 5 minutes.
2. While cooling, set up your steam seat. This can look like a chair without a solid seat (like an outdoor metal chair, or lawn chair), a stool with the center cut out of it, or you can even craft yourself a special vaginal steam box, which looks like a box with a hole cut out of the top. In general, you need a seat to sit on that has holes for the steam to rise up through.
3. Place herbs in water and gently stir (make sure it is still hot enough to produce steam).
4. Place the pot underneath chair.
5. Sit on chair with a bare bottom. Be sure the steam is not so hot it burns your skin.
6. You can either use a large skirt or blankets to cover and wrap yourself. Completely contain the steam within the blanket. You want to create a 'balloon' which directs the steam up through

the top of the chair. Be sure to close any gaps through which the steam can escape.

7. Relax and feel the steam washing your vagina and lower half. While it may not feel like it, the steam is entering into your vagina and moving up to the cervix. Trust that this is happening.
8. Sit for 15-30 minutes. No more, no less.
9. Continue to replenish with hot water if the water goes cool.

You've just vaginal steamed!

Vaginal Douche:

Douching gets a bad rap in many health-circles, yet it is a perfect way to get helping herbs **directly** onto the cervix. While it may be a little awkward at first, washing your cervix in these herbs will greatly support the cervix to self-heal.
I recommend douching 2-3 times a month for Women with a cervical dysplasia/HPV diagnosis.

Vaginal douche herbs:

Ø Goldenseal powder (purchased from a good source as this herb is considered endangered)

Ø Pau d'Arco

Ø Marigold

How to douche:

1. Purchase a douche bulb from your local drug store.

115

2. Fill the bulb with a warm tea using selected herbs. If you are using Goldenseal powder, place 1 tsp. of powder in bulb and fill with warm water. Cover and shake up bulb to mix contents.
3. Douche in shower.
4. *Gently* insert douche stem into the vagina.
    a. I recommend talking with your body and letting her know what you are about to do. Open communication is imperative for self-healing.
5. *Gently* squeeze the bulb. You may need to squeeze it a few times to get all the liquid out.
6. Most of the liquid will fall out of the vagina and down your legs. This is why you do it in the shower.
7. Your cervix has now been washed in healing herbs! It can stay in there, on your cervix, for 1-2 weeks.

*Note: If you are going to the Ob/Gyn to have a pap-test and you have douched, let your doctor know. The herbs may leave your cervix with a strange color (goldenseal turns green while inside — which is totally normal). Unless your doctor knows beforehand, they may be alarmed by what they see. Let them know that you have been doing self-care in order to self-heal.

Essential Oils:

Another way you can incorporate herbal medicine into your Cervical Self Care is through the use of essential oils. An essential oil is a concentrated liquid containing the volatile (or active) aroma compounds of a plant. They are, in essence, the oil of the plant.

You can use essential oils in vaginal suppositories (recipe in self-care ritual tool kit) or placed on tampons to bring the healing compounds close to the cervix. Tampons can be soaked in Protec (a diluted oil combination) with about 4-5 drops of essential oils added, to be inserted vaginally and worn overnight.

Essential oils to use are:

Ø Rosemary

Ø Lemon

Ø Lemongrass

Ø Frankincense

Ø Myrrh

Herbal Body Oiling:

Rubbing oil infused with whole plants is the ultimate self-love ritual. Not only does the fat from the oil penetrate your skin and nourish your nervous system, the entirety of the medicine of the plant is able to penetrate as well. The essential oils and the spiritual essence of the plant are transferred into your bloodstream via the absorption of the oil.

It's important to make sure you purchase herbal body oil that's organic and made with organic plant matter. Given that the skin is the body's largest organ, it's important for you to only put top-quality products on it.

Herbal body oiling does not address HPV and cervical dysplasia directly, but rather supports the body's regeneration through reducing stress. The act of rubbing medicinal oil over your entire body on a daily basis triggers the parasympathetic nervous system and allows the body to relax. Relaxation = regeneration.

Supplements:

Sometimes we just need something easy to do to support our cervical and immune health. This easy street can be found in the form of supplements. Cervical dysplasia has been thought to be related to nutritional deficiencies, including folate, vitamins, A, D, E, and B-vitamins, and trace minerals. Taking a daily multivitamin containing antioxidant vitamins A, C, D, and E, the B-vitamins including folic acid, and trace minerals such as magnesium, calcium, zinc, and selenium can be taken to make sure you are meeting your daily nutritional requirement.

Another supplement I recommend to all my clients is DIM. DIM is a clinically proven supplement which supports the healing and reversal of cervical dysplasia. Oral diindolylmethane (DIM) was found to be effective in the treatment of CIN 2 or 3 lesions on the cervix and was developed to prevent the need for the loop electrosurgical excision procedure (LEEP). This supplement, when purchased as 'bioavailable' from Nature's Way or Enzymatic Therapy, is more effective than folic acid/folate, and makes the beneficial aspects of cruciferous vegetables bioavailable for the body to uptake.[14]

If you do not want to take a multivitamin, these are the various supplements I recommend taking:

Ø Folate

o This supplement was recommended to me by a Naturopathic Doctor. I learned from her that folate strengthens the cell walls, preventing virus' from injecting its DNA in the cell and prohibiting the virus from replicating.

Ø Zinc

Ø Selenium

118

o This trace mineral is found in Brazil nuts. If you eat three brazil nuts a day, you will receive your daily quotient of selenium.

Ø Lysine

Ø B Vitamins

*Disclaimer: I do not recommend purchasing all of the above supplements and taking them without consulting your doctor or physician. Choose one or two which resonate and start there. Also, *do not* purchase the cheapest supplements. If you choose to take supplements to support your healing journey, do yourself a favor and invest in high-quality supplements. Many supplements have fillers and sugar in them. Do a little research on your own about brands and whether or not the supplement contains anything else than what the label says.

Stop Smoking Tobacco:

If you smoke tobacco and have HPV and a cervical dysplasia diagnosis, I highly advocate and invite you to STOP. Smoking tobacco is directly linked to a reduction of immune function and an increase in cervical cancer. According to the CDC, Women who smoke are 3 times more likely to develop cervical cancer. This is also true for Women who are around second-hand smoke.[16] It is crucial for you to cease smoking cigarettes and remove yourself from any location that has polluted air caused by cigarette smoke.

Exposure to pollutants and carcinogens (such as cigarette smoke) inhibits the body's immune system and allows for HPV and cell abnormalities to proliferate.

If you are having a difficult time stopping smoking, I invite you to reach out to someone. Find a support system as you work through the stages of addiction recovery. There is no shame in admitting to having difficulty in smoking cessation. You're not alone. There is compassion for those who try to change and come up against roadblocks. It's a large part of being human.

Transition off Hormonal Birth Control:

According to the Center for Disease Control website, research shows that long-term use (5+ years) of oral contraceptives (birth control pills) creates a nearly threefold increase in the risk of cervical cancer (what cervical dysplasia may lead to if left untreated). For Women who have used oral contraceptives for ten years or longer, the risk of cervical cancer is **four times higher**.[17]

You may be wondering, though, just how exogenous hormones (hormones from outside our own body) can lead to an increased prevalence of cervical cancer.

In a 2008 study, researchers found that having an excess of estrogen in our body synergizes with an increase in HPV oncogenes (a gene that has the potential to cause cancer).[18] The cervix is highly responsive to estrogen, and the hormones found in oral contraceptives change the susceptibility of cervical cells to HPV infection. This, then, affects the cell's ability to clear the infection, ultimately leading to abnormalities in the cervical cells.

If you've been diagnosed with cervical dysplasia and/or HPV, it is best to transition off of exogenous hormones to bring balance back to the body's endocrine system. Other hormonal birth control options (IUD, implants, NuvaRing, etc.) use the same hormones as the pill (progestin and estrogen). If you are using these forms of contraception, it may be wise to transition as well. Non-hormonal options include condoms (male or female), diaphragms, copper IUDs, and the Fertility Awareness Method/ Fertility tracking (which you can find resources in the Resources section). It is your decision how you want to keep yourself from unwanted pregnancy. I simply want you to be informed as to how hormonal birth control affects cervical wellness.

It is also important to keep the number of new sexual partners low. This follows the logic that the more sexual partners one has, the greater the risk of exposure to strains of HPV and the higher the chance of prolonged cervical dysplasia. Feel free to explore your sexuality, just keep in mind clear communication regarding past partners/STI testing, and use barrier-forms of contraceptives.

Spend Time Outside, In Nature, As Often as You Can:

It is well known that spending time outside has positive benefits on overall health and wellness. Spending intentional time out in nature is especially important, valuable and vital for Women's reproductive health.

Women are representative of Earth. We're life-producing, and as such, have an inherent connection to the Earth and to nature. While there's little clinical scientific data to support specifically the benefits to Women's health at this time, I'll share with you four reasons why I believe spending time in nature needs to be an aspect of a Woman's self-care regimen.

1. *Phytoncides*

Phytoncides are volatile essential oils emitted by plants and trees which have been proven to increase immune function within adults.[19] These oils boost the activity of natural killer cells of the immune system, which are especially important in the journey of healing HPV and

121

cervical dysplasia. Natural killer cells search and destroy virus and cancerous cells before they're able to multiply.

One highly effective way to boost the immune functioning of the body is to spend thirty minutes once a week in an outdoor (ideally wild) environment, inhaling these volatile essential oil compounds. A thirty-minute experience of inhaling air with phytoncides boosts immune functioning for up to one week. Getting a weekly dose of nature-air will help keep your immune system strong and functioning at top strength.

2. *Provides perspective on the cyclical nature of the Feminine:*

Western culture is hyper-focused on growth and linear perspectives (both of which are traditional 'masculine' traits), and many Women struggle with adapting to this. We see many Women attempting to 'be' like Men, and this is detrimental to the ways in which they associate with their own cyclical reproductive nature. Many women feel shameful, adverse or flat-out resistant to the ways in which their bodies function, and this can be amended by making intentional contact with nature.

The reproductive workings of a Woman actually mirror that of nature — holding the primordial codes of Life and Death within its own cyclical nature. Just like Earth has seasons, a Woman's body cycles through seasons of its own on a monthly basis through the menstruation/ovulation cycle.

When we experience Earth's seasons out in nature, we begin to find a deep internal acceptance to our own cyclical nature. We are able to notice how our own body is akin to that of Earth and a greater sense of acceptance, connection and love is established for our body. Perhaps there will be less striving to be more 'masculine' and our inherent 'feminine' nature will emerge once women accept that their bodies are akin to the nature of the Earth.

3. Bleeding on the Earth

Earth and humans (and all life for that matter) have bioelectric fields. We all have bioelectricity running through us, just as Earth has bioelectricity running through it as well.

It's commonly known that water, especially saltwater, is electrically conductive; meaning, electricity can travel through it easily. Menstrual blood is made up largely of water, and contains sodium as well. When a Woman bleeds directly onto the Earth, the menstrual blood creates a perfect bridge between her body's and Earth's electrical fields.

The Earth electrically resonates at roughly 7.83 Hz. This is the ideal resonance for humans as well, yet with the advent of modern technologies such as rubber-soled shoes, plastic, laminate, WIFI, skyscrapers and cars, humans have become disconnected from this electrical resonance. This disconnection has led to imbalanced human electrical systems. The electrical system of our body is the nervous system. When the nervous system is out of balance, anxiety, depression, fatigue, stress, and disease become more prevalent.

There's a movement called Earthing that is growing in popularity throughout the world. Earthing is based upon the discovery that connecting to Earth's natural (bioelectric) energy is foundational for whole-human health. Earthing is essentially placing your bare feet/arms/whole body onto uncovered Earth, such as grass, the beach, soil, or wild, running water. This direct connection gives the human body a charge of bioelectric energy and 'dumps' excess electric charge out of our system, helping us to feel better and more balanced.

Bleeding directly onto the Earth is the *ultimate* Earthing. Not only does a Woman receive the benefits of simply sitting on the Earth, but the blood directs Earth's energy directly into her womb, providing her 'female generative battery' an opportunity to come back into resonance with the Earth. Earth's energy enters into the body via the vaginal canal and flows into the uterus via the blood coming out through the cervix. Pouring more energy into this part of a Woman's body is like charging her creative/spiritual battery. The uterus/womb is the creative/generative center of the female body, and providing this location with a dose of Earth's energy helps to recharge this location in our architecture.

The Cervix is the sacred doorway for the connection of Earth to penetrate a Woman's womb. Bleeding directly on the Earth is one of the most potent ways to connect to Cervix, to Earth, and to the Womb. It is the Spiritual Gas-Station that so many women need today. This method of nature connection (Women sitting on the Earth while menstruating) has been recorded throughout time, and it is time that modern Women adopt these old ways once again. Bleeding directly on the Earth can help with mental problems, fatigue, cervical problems, and self-esteem. I highly encourage and invite all Women to try this practice at least once.

10 Steps to Bleed on the Earth

*I recommend doing this within the first three days of your cycle, when it is the heaviest

1. Find a relatively secluded area outside. If not secluded, that is okay.
2. Wear a big skirt, dress, robe, blanket, or towel outside
3. Take off your underwear. Do not have a tampon or cup in. Use no pad or anything else to stop your flow.
4. With the skirt/dress/robe belled out, or with the towel/blanket wrapped around your waist, take a seat on the earth — with nothing underneath you.
5. I recommend a patch of grass or clover. If you are sitting on dirt/sand, dig a little pocket to sit over. You don't want the Yoni to get too dirty.
6. Sit. Breathe. Feel. (For me, as soon as I sit down on the Earth, my body releases blood like it was waiting for the connection. Don't be surprised if you feel a 'gush').
7. I invite you to sit there for at least 20 minutes. Journal. Meditate. Breathe. Enjoy the nature surroundings. Have a friend bleeding too? Have her join!
8. Once you feel complete, put your underwear back on and stand up.
9. Look at the blood you released onto the Earth. Gaze at its beauty, and acknowledge its offering. You have completed the cycle, returning 'what could have been' back to the Earth.
10. Notice how you feel. Is there a difference in your felt-sensations in your body after bleeding on the Earth? Notice any subtle changes or shifts. This is a sacred connection you've just made.

I'd like to end this section by stating that the way in which the biosphere of our planet is treated is very much the way in which Women's bodies are treated. Just like the 'natural resources' of our planet, Women's bodies are commodified, legislated on, assaulted and extracted from without permission or consent.

Spending time in nature will not only improve the overall physical, mental and emotional health of a Woman of reproductive age, but it will bolster her ability to stand true in her power as a person who encompasses the Life-Death-Rebirth qualities of our great planet. Given the political climate of today, this is increasingly needed.

And so, if you are a Woman of reproductive age, I implore you — go outside, spend as much time in nature as you can, and recognize the power that you hold as an embodiment of Earth. It is high time we live up to this fact.

4. *Sexual Habit Awareness and Cervical Literacy*

Sex. It is one of the most primal actions we as humans can make. The impulse to have sex, alongside eating and sleeping, is rooted deep within our brain and body. Our body sends off chemicals called pheromones to attract potential sexual partners. Multiple organ systems are wired to support the process of having sex, including our nervous, cardiovascular and endocrine systems. We are pleasure-seeking animals who go out of our way to feel pleasure in our bodies from sexual stimulation. Sex is a part of being human. Unfortunately, for most Americans today, the way we've learned about sex and sexual intimacy has come from sources that tend to skip over female-body literacy and pleasure.

For many modern adults, their knowledge of sex has come from pornography and the public sex-education system, both of which fail to portray the intricacies of the female sexual responses of arousal and pleasure. Cis-hetero pornography tends to be male-centered, with the female body portrayed as an object of desire and pleasure for the male. These images are compounded by the fact that Western marketing tactics exemplify this story, as well. Contemporary sex education in the public-school system is focused on abstinence, basic reproduction physiology, and birth control. There is never any mention of pleasure and pain, emotional literacy, consent, nor the necessity of foreplay. This is highly unfortunate for those with female bodies.

Most female-bodied people haven't been told that it is okay to speak up in advocacy for their bodies during sex. We've been conditioned that we're supposed to acquiesce to whatever is done to us in the bedroom, and that pain is a (normal) part of the experience. Think about how often we hear that losing our virginity is expected to be painful. This is a common story young women are told about their sexual experience. We're also made to believe that our pleasure comes second to the males' and that as soon as he has his climax, the whole experience ends. We're fearful that if we speak up, should we feel pain, our partner will get upset and reject us. These sexual patterns are unhealthy and unbalanced. They lead to women feeling/being closed-off to sexual pleasure and simply 'going through the motions' without receiving the benefits.

Women are inherent 'givers' and many times engage in sexual activities for the sake of their partner, rather than because they are feeling turned on. Unfortunately, the choice to continue with sexual intercourse when there is no desire or when pain is present is harmful to cervical health. A woman should never make love unless she truly wants to, for the action of penetrative sex without adequate desire can be traumatizing to a woman's body.

Pain during sex is your cervix crying out to be seen and heard. The cervix wants whatever is coming into contact with it to stop. When a woman is leading her daily life, the cervix sits fairly low in the vagina

— roughly 2-4 inches from the opening. The uterus is tilted forward in the body cavity and there isn't much extra 'space' for anything else to enter in. Yet when a woman becomes aroused, the brain sends signals to the body, informing it that it wants to be penetrated. The uterus tilts back into the body to make space and the cervix *moves up and out of the way*. The body *literally* creates space inside the vaginal canal for whatever is going to be penetrating. The vaginal canal opens and elongates between 6-8 inches. This physiological mechanism places the cervix at the perfect position to be out of the way of harm while simultaneously in the perfect position to receive pleasure.

Unfortunately, many Women don't have the opportunity to experience this opening and pleasure. For many, their sexual experiences are rushed, and time isn't provided for the body to send all the signals and to slowly open. The imagery of a flower blooming is a wonderful metaphor for this internal experience. You can't rush a flower blooming, just like you can't rush the female body into opening more quickly than it is able.

Most women I speak to can relate to this experience of feeling a phallus 'hit the end', or that dull internal thumping feeling causing pain during penetration. That feeling is an indication that there was not enough time to make space and for opening to occur. That pain is your cervix being hit.

"Problems with a woman's sexual organs are often related to her inability to say no to penetration when she wants to but does not think she should."
-Dr. Christiane Northrup, MD

This quote by Dr. Christiane Northrup sums this up so clearly. Saying yes to penetration even though your body is not yet ready can damage the delicate transformation zone of the cervix. The pain felt in the body leads to micro-traumas which may cause the cells in the transformation zone to rescind and recoil — trying to protect themselves from being hit and feeling pain. Waiting for penetration until properly aroused is for the safety of our body. This allows time for the cervix to move up and into the body cavity, elongating the vaginal canal and making space for penetration. If you feel pain during sex, this is your cervix saying "No! I'm not ready!"

Cervical dysplasia can be seen as an 'armoring' of the cervix. When you grit and bear through painful sex, you're intentionally silencing the voice of your body. You're numbing out. This conscious choice to not listen to the cervix leads your body to believe you're not with her, and so she responds. She's crying out for help because she wants pleasure and penetration, but only when she is ready.

You're worthy of pleasure. Your needs are valid and important. Finding the courage within you to express your needs in sex opens up the vagus nerve pathway, stimulates your parasympathetic nervous system, and allows your body to relax.

If any of this resonates with you, begin to reflect on when and how often you engage in sex when you don't feel like it or aren't ready. Talk to your partner or find support from friends. This is an important step of self-reflection to reconnect to your cervix and body, and to hear whether or not you have been listening to their needs. Develop a self-love practice that includes only engaging in sexual activities when you really desire to.

Using your voice during sex in order to protect your cervix from future damage is one of the main takeaways I want you to remember from this book. By becoming our body's #1 advocate, we can deepen our connection and relationship to it. When we engage in sex without proper arousal, we're putting our cervix at risk of being damaged and harmed. We *must* have our body's back if we want to heal.

In summary...

All of the self-care tools and tips mentioned are ways in which you can begin to connect and tend to your cervix. Combining these tools and tips with healthy lifestyle and wellness practices will guide your body to return to its vital, natural state. Everything I've shared here is manageable and can be incorporated into your daily life.

There are more resources and tools in the Self Care and Ritual Toolkit, which can be found in subsequent sections. These resources come from past clients who've tried them out and found success. I did not make them a large part of the book because I personally have not experienced them. I offer them to you to include in your own exploration journey.

I invite you to take one step at a time and not to overload yourself all at once. Begin with one practice or tool, do that for a while, and then incorporate another practice or tip. Slowly build up your stamina with transforming your life to meet the needs of your body and cervix so that they can heal.

Do not try to do everything at once — you will overload yourself and then you won't wish to try anymore. Be gentle and caring. Go with what feels right. Our body is relearning how to take care of itself, and we must take small, baby-steps to integrate this knowing.

If a practice or tool doesn't work for you, *you don't have to do it.* Allow your body and cervix to guide you to what it needs in order to heal. This method of taking care of cervical dysplasia (or preventing it) takes time, but it is long lasting.

You are worthy of taking care of your body and your cervix. Your cervix and body are 110% worth all the changes that need to be made so you can heal.

Once again, I want to remind you, that if you have been diagnosed with HPV and cervical dysplasia, to be kind and compassionate to yourself. Recognize that the choices you've made in the past have gotten you to where you are, but you can now make new and informed decisions for the love and support of your cervix, your reproductive system, and your whole body. This book provides tools and resources to begin your healing journey, but I encourage you to explore options for yourself. I encourage you to take on the role as the expert of your body and experience, and to trust that your body is constantly wanting to achieve a state of balance and wellness.

PART FOUR
PROBLEMS WITH MODERN GYNECOLOGY

CHAPTER SEVEN
PROBLEMS WITH MODERN GYNECOLOGY

MEDICAL gynecology is wonderful for certain things. This field of medicine is very proficient in helping Women in chronic and acute reproductive-situations, and the advent of new technologies and preventative testing has saved many lives. Without modern gynecology, thousands of Women would experience prolonged discomfort and distress (and even death) from a wide range of acute conditions including eclampsia, vaginal fistulas, breech births, hemorrhage, and ruptured ovarian cysts.

However, regardless of the benefits of modern gynecology, there are several aspects of this medical field I see as problematic and potentially dangerous. I explain three of these aspects here.

LACK OF INFORMATION OFFERED

THERE exists a generalized global trend of Women not receiving proper education and information surrounding their gynecological, reproductive and sexual health. It amazes me how many Women don't know what is being checked during a pap test or why they even need to care. We obediently go to have exams, tests and procedures done without knowing the real reasons why we need to go in the first place.

Contemporary public sex education and reproductive literacy programs are devoid of information on some of the most important and valuable subjects – like the cervix. When I think back to the sex education I received in middle and high school, I don't remember them speaking on the cervix other than when commenting on birth and cervical dilation. The cervix wasn't even mentioned when I went in to receive my first pap smear. I only went in because I was told I need one by the nice lady at Planned Parenthood when I snuck there to get birth control pills at the age of fifteen. I literally had no idea what was happening or why.

This is a problem. Women are walking into medical offices completely uninformed about what is actually going on in their bodies. When medical professionals use words and language we are unfamiliar with, many of us feign knowledge so as to not be made to look ignorant. We pretend to understand, when in reality we don't.

When a Woman does not have all the necessary information, she cannot make informed decisions. When we can't make informed decisions, we don't feel empowered in the experience. We place our power into the hands of someone else who *seems* to know more than we do. This handing over of power has left many Women saying yes to treatment options they didn't actually want, while feeling resentful that they weren't told more.

Having Women blindly make decisions based upon what their medical practitioner says is dangerous and immoral. This is especially true for women whom are young adults (18-23 yrs. old) and who may not have had much life experience yet.

We need to be told exactly what is happening and why. We need to be explained clearly what the potential consequences of going through the surgical procedures are (read: numb cervix, difficulty in future childbirth, no guarantee of success), and what the side effects are of the vaccines. If these are the only treatments available via Western medicine, then it is the responsibility of the medical practitioners to provide information and the responsibility of the patient to ask questions.

LIMITED OPTIONS FOR HELP AND SUPPORT

W HEN a Woman receives an abnormal pap-test result, the first thing that comes to her mind is, 'Well, what can I do?'

In Cervical Wellness, we talk about the lifestyle and habit changes that can be made to help the body heal naturally. We offer various tools, methods, tips, tricks and perspectives to use in supporting the cervix to heal HPV and cervical dysplasia, and work to give options for people of all lifestyles.

Western medicine provides two types of options: surgery or vaccination. We can get the face of their cervix burned/frozen or surgically removed, or we can opt-in to receive the HPV vaccine (though I have never understood why one would opt-in for a vaccine for something already present). That is it. There are no other options for help and support with HPV and cervical dysplasia.

These two categories of options are limited. There is no availability for guidance and support of an individual to adopt the changes she needs to make in order to allow her body to heal on its own (which it is quite capable of doing). There are only options to remove the afflicted cells from the body in the *hope* that it will not return, or to vaccinate against a virus the body is already working with.

This is a major problem.

When a Woman feels anxious and fearful upon receiving the abnormal test result, she tends go to the first thing that is offered by her medical practitioner, because she wants it gone. I've received hundreds of stories of Women approaching their doctor, asking them what they can do to help, and the doctors tell them about the LEEP procedure. With no other options present, she goes through it, has a terrible time, searches the internet, discovers there are other ways, and then feels immense grief over the fact that her doctor allowed her to get surgery when there were other choices. I have had many women send me messages like, 'I feel like it is too late. I went with the LEEP and I wish I had known there were other ways.'

There are other ways. Yes, the surgeries are a perfect option for *some people*. But to offer them to *every* person with *all grades* of cervical dysplasia is barbaric and unnecessary. Someone who has CIN I does not need the same treatment as someone with CIN III or carcinoma in-situ. Placing everyone under the umbrella of limited treatment options does not take into account their individual lifestyle, their history, their mindset and perspective, and their beliefs-system.

There needs to be a broader conversation of what leads to cervical dysplasia so that all women understand what aspects of lifestyle play into the health of the cervix. Treatment options should include education and guidance around non-invasive methods of treating HPV and cervical dysplasia. It's time to make this so.

POSITION OF
DISEMPOWERMENT

GYNECOLOGICAL exams are some of the most intrusive, boundary-crossing types of physical exams there are (in my opinion). In these exams, we are subject to exposing the most vulnerable part of our body, penetrated by foreign objects, and swabbed and scraped in our innermost sanctum. These exams are not comfortable for anyone.

Many Women feel nervous and anxious when their pap-test is approaching. The idea of going through the process can be distressing, and many people endure extreme emotional discomfort. Some choose to opt-out and not go through the exam because of this discomfort. Once in the doctor's office, they may feel even more nervous, anxious, or even numbed to the whole experience (for self-preservation). They just want to get through it.

While in this mind-state, we are then required to lie on their back, put our feet in stirrups and then spread our legs wide for the exam. The table is propped up high so as to put the doctor or nurse practitioner in a comfortable position to do the exam. This position puts us further into a state of helplessness.

Lying on our backs with our legs spread is one of the most vulnerable positions a human can put themselves in. It is the position

141

of ultimate submission. It is the complete surrender of the power of the body.

I see putting Women in this position as one of the key major problems with modern gynecology. In my research into the history of gynecology and Women's health, I have come across dozens of images of midwives and medical practitioners treating women in a completely different way than that to which we're all now so accustomed.

In each of these images, what is clear is that the patient's comfort is held as the most important. The Woman is sitting in a chair, supported by other Women. The midwife is seated or kneeling on the ground, below the individual who is seated in the chair. There are no stirrups. The patient is not elevated on a table, open and exposed to the whole room. There is decency. There is dignity.

On the other hand, in modern gynecology we're presented with a lack of dignity. Yes, we are given medical gowns to wear so that we aren't completely exposed. Yes, the medical practitioners are trained in ethical practices and have taken the Hippocratic Oath to do no harm. Yes, the intention of OB/GYN practitioners is to help and be of service. All of this is true.

Yet, there is still a problem. Women still feel disempowered in their gynecological experiences, and the physical position we are placed in during these experiences plays into these feelings.

As a historian, I am deeply interested in learning the 'why' of things. Why are we placed in this position? Why is this the way exams are done nowadays? This seems very different than the way female-bodies were treated in the past. What happened?

CHAPTER EIGHT
A HISTORY OF DISEMPOWERMENT

MANY Women have stories of uncomfortable experiences during gynecological appointments. The vulnerable feeling of lying on your back, legs spread wide, feet in stirrups, opened for the whole world to see is one that many Women lament about. There is nothing empowering about this position.

Females are poked, prodded, scraped, and swabbed inside their most delicate area, and discomfort is assumed — normalized, even. In today's Western medical model, these sorts of practices are common and considered a necessary part of any Woman's health regimen. Many assume that it's "just how it is done".

However, much of the history of modern medicine has a shadow-side; a dark background wherein methods and practices once seen as barbaric and negative have transformed into everyday occurrences. What follows is a brief history of two aspects of modern gynecology. I share this to inform Women of the background of these 'modern' practices.

It is important to know where we come from in order to inform where we are going. The history of contemporary gynecological practices suggests a lack of value placed in Women's health-empowerment, and I hope that through reading this story, a fire is ignited in you to reclaim your dignity as a female, and to be in charge of your gynecological health to the best of your ability.

THE 'FATHER' OF MODERN GYNECOLOGY

J AMES Marion Sims (1813-
1870) is nationally recognized
as the "Father of
Gynecology". Sims was an
American physician and
surgeon who pioneered the
surgical intervention for the
repair of vesicovaginal fistula,
a complication of obstructed
childbirth. This complication
causes women to constantly
leak urine into the vagina due
to a tear between the bladder
and vagina. During Sims' era,
Women with this complication
were considered outcasts of society.

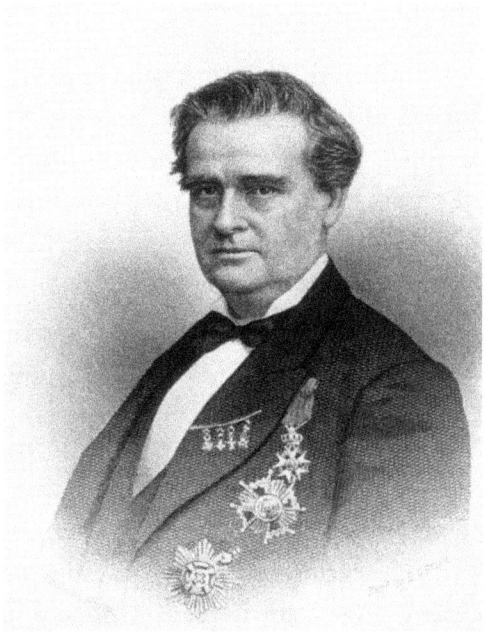

In order to perfect his surgical techniques, Sims used black slave
Women as experimental test subjects. Without the use of any anesthesia
or numbing, Sims practiced his examinations and surgical interventions.
Betsy, Lucy and Anarcha were three of the Women used in his

experimental procedures. Anarcha had thirty separate surgeries, all without anesthesia.

Throughout his experimentation, Sims developed procedures, methods, and tools which allowed him easier access to a Women's interior vaginal canal. He is the noted inventor of the speculum, the use of stirrups (which were originally used to hold the patient down without moving), and the exposed position of the patient on the table. Once Sims perfected his procedures, he then began practice on white patients — albeit with anesthesia.

Today's Influence

James Marion Sims is regarded as a medical hero, and is honored for his addition to medical knowledge in the realm of pelvic surgery for Women. At the time of the first version of this book, there was a statue of him in his honor in North Carolina and Central Park, NYC; the latter having since been removed and placed in the cemetery where he is buried. The removal of the statue was inspired and fueled by the Black Lives Matter movement in 2018.

I am not here to denounce Sims or say that his honoring should be revoked. His methods have helped many Women who suffer from vesicovaginal fistula and has transformed the way gynecological surgery was originally viewed. However, I am here to question the tactics used to treat these patients and the continuation of the use of extremely disempowering tools such as stirrups and insertion of the speculum before a Woman is ready (which routinely over-stretches and causes many women physical and psychological discomfort).

I understand that medical professionals must be able to see the inside of the vaginal canal and cervix for health reasons, but why not make the methods and procedure more comfortable? More cozy, sacred and dare I say, pleasurable. I question the insertion of the speculum

146

without allowing the Woman to take a few deep breaths to prepare herself for penetration. I wonder why mirrors are not offered regularly so Women may participate in the exam, rather than merely be subjected to it. Why, I wonder, are we treating modern-day gynecology patients in the same methods and with the same mannerisms that were used to treat unwilling experimental patients? These questions and thoughts propel this book.

THE COLPOSCOPY

WESTERN medicine is full of procedures and treatments that people do not question. There is no inquiry into the root of said procedures and treatments, and it is assumed that this is the only way it can be done as it is the way it's currently done. This is most true for the colposcopy.

For all those who have had a colposcopy, you know what it is. There is no way to ever forget what one is. For all those who have not had a colposcopy, I will explain what it is here.

The exact definition of a colposcopy is "a medical diagnostic procedure to examine an illuminated view of the cervix and the tissues of the vagina and vulva... It is done using a colposcope, which provides an enlarged view of the areas, allowing the colposcopist to visually distinguish normal from abnormal appearing tissue and take directed biopsies for further pathological examination." [25] Colposcopies are administered during a follow-up appointment, following abnormal pap test results. Colposcopies help to determine the level of cervical dysplasia present, and can assess its grade (CIN I/II/III).

What is most felt and experienced by the patient are the biopsies taken during the examination. These are what make colposcopies so painfully memorable for so many. The biopsies are taken without anesthesia or numbing. For many, these biopsies are painful and

148

traumatic, especially when multiple colposcopies are needed over the course of several months.

Throughout my entire healing journey and all the colpos I received, I never questioned them. I was made to believe that it was normal to experience extreme pain/pinching and subsequent bleeding of my cervix in order to heal myself, and as such went along with receiving them. I remember my doctor explaining the colposcopy as a 'hole punch' of the cervix. Hearing the phrase 'hole punch' and thinking about it taking a piece of my body didn't ever settle well with me, yet I never questioned it.

It wasn't until much later, when I was sharing about the history of James Marion Sims, that I learned about the dark history of colposcopies through a client. Upon diving into the history of this routine procedure, it all became clear.

The colposcopy procedure and colposcope was developed in the early twentieth century by the prestigious German physician and professor Hans Hinselmann as a way to make an examination of the cervix easier. In Western gynecology at this time, viewing the cervix was difficult because of the distance of focus. Hinselmann tried to solve this problem by pulling out the uterine cervix with forceps, but this only caused immense pain to the patient. In response, Hinselmann invented the colposcope and biopsy procedure but did not have any Women to practice or experiment on.

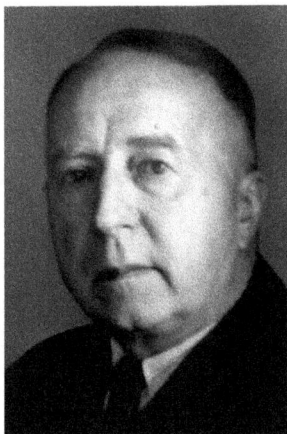

In the early 1940s, Hinselmann found support from Eduard Wirths, the chief camp physician for the notorious Jewish "medical block 10" of Auschwitz concentration camp, whom offered him a place to test his newly invented procedure and viewing device. These medical experiments involved Jewish inmates in Auschwitz.[26]

Hinselmann performed his medical experiments on unwilling prisoners of war in German concentration camps. The Women were subject to painful and lengthy procedures on their cervix as the camp's medical doctors attempted to figure out a way to get a better look and take biopsies.

What became clear when I learned about the history of this procedure is that this form of examination and treatment in no way takes into consideration the felt- and lived-experience of the patient herself. In fact, the Women who were used to 'perfect' this technique were deemed below human, and as such, pain and discomfort were not taken into account.

A STARK REALITY

T HE root of the most common practices and procedures of modern gynecology are buried in a history of experimental slavery. There is a deep well of disturbing harm that was caused, all in the name of 'good' and 'medicine'. Throughout the development of these practices, the emotional safety, pain threshold, and body-autonomy of Women were lost. I bring into question these practices that do not honor female bodies and instead have only used them as a means to an end.

Both of these men have been touted as medical heroes in Western medicine. Their advancements changed the course of gynecology and are routinely used today. I often wonder about the 'root of harm' and how so many women come out of the gynecological exam room feeling worse than when they entered. There is an air surrounding these commonplace practices, and with the revealing of this history, it is clear that it is a feeling of malevolence.

I do not think people who are practicing gynecology are malevolent. I know those who choose to enter into the field of medicine do so because they want to be of service and to help others. It is an act of selflessness to devote your life to medicine: I recognize this.

Regardless of the altruism that many medical doctors feel, this does not negate the stark reality that the practices and procedures they perform daily are rooted in a mindset that is against the female form.

Their perspective on the ability for Women to speak the truth of their pain and discomfort are colored by what the medical texts say. A male-doctor performing a colposcopy could in no way understand what it is like to have a 'hole-punch' taken to one of their most sensitive body parts, yet because the literature describes it as only a 'pinch', they feel no cause for concern.

A CALL FOR PATIENT-EMPOWERMENT IN GYNECOLOGY

ALL those with a female body want to be healthy. They want their reproductive organs to be healthy and function well, and they want to make sure that everything is OK 'down there'. We also want to be involved in this process; only, there just doesn't seem to be any room for them to be so. I'm bringing into question the current status quo of placing the comfort of the doctor in higher regard than the comfort of the patient, and I am calling for a reworking of the way in which a 'closer look' is performed.

Why can't the doctor be squatting or sitting lower than the table with the woman standing or crouching herself; rather than being on her back, spread-eagle? Why can't the patient determine how far the speculum stretches, or how quickly it opens her up, allowing the body to gradually get used to the notion of being so exposed? Why can't the patient insert the speculum themselves, allowing them the time and space to open to penetration, as well as a more direct advocacy over their own bodies? Why isn't there another way to determine what grade cervical dysplasia is without taking multiple biopsies? How come innovation of these gynecological practices and procedures stopped with Sims and Hinselmann? Why aren't we working towards developing practices and procedures that put the comfort and felt-experience of the Woman as top priority? These are only some of the questions I hold, and the list continues to grow.

A way to counteract the current of disempowerment in a gynecological exam and procedure is to use your own voice in advocacy of your body. For the first time in 2,000+ years, Women have the opportunity to speak out and stand up for themselves in the name of their health and healing. Right now, Women have more freedom to use their voice in advocacy and self-preservation than any other time over the past millennia. I invite and encourage you to speak up about feelings of discomfort or pain. Use your voice and tell your doctor if you are not ready for penetration. *They are there to serve you; not the other way around.* You are in control of what happens to your body, and unless you reserve that power for yourself, practitioners may do that for you.

I invite and encourage you to take a moment to breathe, center in your body, and remind your body that you love her and that, although you find yourself in this compromising position, you have the power because you are choosing to show up. Remember, it is your body and you have the ultimate say as to what happens to it, even while in a medical appointment.

It's time to reclaim your power in gynecology.

CHAPTER NINE

ENERGETICS OF A MOVEMENT:

#metoo AND #timesup

WHEN I began work with Cervical Wellness, I had no idea the implications of what I was bringing to the world. Asking Women to connect to this body part that has endured millennia of pain and trauma brought so much up to the surface that I feared I had done something wrong. Through the process of connecting to their cervixes, my clients remembered experiences they had originally repressed or wanted to forget. Often times, the pain that wells up from this remembrance can be overwhelming, to say the least.

In Cervical Wellness, I teach that all the memories of everything that has ever penetrated you (physical or energetic) are remembered by the Cervix. The cervix is the place in the body that comes into direct contact with whatever penetrates. This is how we can become energetically tethered/codependent with another. It's scary to think how many Women are energetically hooked by Men they do not want to be attached to, and that this is unconsciously affecting their everyday lives. It's even scarier to think about how many Women have experienced forced penetration on a physical level as well. Rape and sexual assault are so prolific that it took a hashtag on social media to bring it to light.

The #metoo movement unleashed the rage of the Cervix.

This social media movement gave Women an opportunity to open up about their experiences with sexual assault, harassment and rape. What drew the media's attention was not the fact that Women were speaking up — there have been Women who were whistleblowers of sexual assault and rape in the past – but rather, the sheer number of

Women who used that hashtag. Millions of Women stepped out of the shame-closet and used their voice in the way they were given permission to: #metoo. On Twitter, the hashtag was reportedly used by 1.7 Million Women in 85 countries [23], and on Facebook the hashtag claimed 12 million posts, comments and reactions within 24 hours [24]. These are no small numbers.

The #metoo movement happened to coincide perfectly with the Harvey Weinstein scandal (where the ex-Miramax film producer had over 80 Women accuse him of sexual misconduct) and the Larry Nassar case (the ex-USA Gymnastics team doctor and osteopathic physician at Michigan State University who was accused by over 100 young women of childhood sexual abuse). More individuals are coming under the spotlight as well, and there are far too many to list here. What needs to be said, however, is that the rage of the cervix is only just beginning to be expressed.

On January 1, 2018, Women of Hollywood created another social medial hashtag in response to the Harvey Weinstein scandal called #timesup (https://www.timesupnow.com/). This hashtag has become the internet war cry of the Cervix. Through these Women, the Voice of the Cervix is rising up and saying, *No more. No more this way. Time is up*! The voice of the cervix has finally been heard and Women around the world are now listening to what our bodies have been crying out for generations: It's time for us to heal and to be sovereign in our body's experience.

This is what I envision this work to be. A starting point for all those with female bodies to reconnect to this place that holds *so much*, to feel it *all*, to process what has been done, to call out who needs to be called out, to forgive who needs to be forgiven, to forgive ourselves, to love ourselves, to touch ourselves, to nurture ourselves, and finally to heal ourselves of what needs to be healed. I truly *know* that cervical dysplasia is the voice of the cervix asking you to pay attention to it; to bring your focus and awareness down to this shadowy body part, so that all of the above can happen.

We do not have to have another #metoo experience. We do not need to be afraid of what stories are hidden in our cervix. #Timesup for the old ways of being. It's time for our Warrior to arise and the Voice of our Cervix to be heard once and for all.

PART FIVE | RESOURCES

CHAPTER TEN
CERVICAL TOOL-KIT

THIS section of the book offers different tools you can draw upon to support you in your healing journey. Some of these tools I developed, some I received from past clients, some I found on my own journey.

I offer them to you as invitations.

Here is what is included in the Tool Kit:

- Cervical Wellness Oath of Self Love and Self-Advocacy
- How to Create an Altar to Support You on Your Healing Journey
- 7 Days of Daily Touch
- Journal Prompts for Self-Inquiry
- Sample Recipes for Cervical Wellness
- Other Goodies and Resources

I want to remind you once more of how healing is a process and a journey, and how it does not serve to do too much at once. I invite you to take one or two steps at a time and allow them to integrate in your body and life. Once you feel them integrated, then you can move into including more in your healing regimen. Doing too much will only overwhelm you and cause you to rebel against the process of healing.

OATH OF SELF-LOVE AND SELF-ADVOCACY

*T*HIS *oath is spoken out loud, every day, in the morning:*

I solemnly swear, in the presence of my Heart, Mind and Higher-Self, to commit to cultivating a loving relationship with my cervix, reproductive system and body.

I choose to put the past behind me and step forward on a new path of awareness and empowerment.

I honor the Voice of my Body and use my own Voice to speak up in advocacy of my body with sexual partners, doctors and even my own Mind.

I allow the hurtful, painful and rejected memories stored within my body to be released with ease and pleasure. Like a snake shedding its old skin, I choose to remove the parts of me that are holding me back from becoming the Woman I know I can become.

I call upon my Higher Self to assist and guide me through the process of allowing that which no longer serves me — mindsets, beliefs, self-

163

judgments, energies and memories — to be cleansed from my Body, and in their place, feelings of acceptance, forgiveness, joy, love and pleasure emerge and are cultivated.

I accept and receive unexpected insights, visions, inspirations, abundance, joy and pleasure.
I choose to unconditionally love myself and to listen to the Voice of my Body.

It is done.
It is done.
It is done.

By the power of three,
In a sacred trinity,
It is done.

CREATING AN ALTAR FOR YOUR CERVICAL WELLNESS JOURNEY

An altar creates a central focus for the energy cultivated and moved throughout your healing journey. Anything can be put on an altar — it doesn't have to be just feathers, stones, and candles (although those are really great things to place on an altar).

There are no 'rules' to creating an altar. It is a creative act of inspiration and devotion.

Steps to creating your altar:

1. Find a place for your altar to be. Next to a window is nice, or somewhere you will see it often. Make it accessible, yet out of the way so that it does not get messed up. Ideally, there will be a piece of furniture where you build your altar. This can be the top of a dresser, a small table, mantle, or even a stool. Any piece of furniture that has a flat top where you are able to view the top while sitting or standing will work.

2. Place a piece of cloth over the top. This will be the base of your altar. Choose a piece of cloth with a color or pattern that feels good and inspiring to you. What colors encourage you to connect to your cervix? What sort of pattern (if any) inspires you to persevere? Sometimes it is nice to purchase a special piece of cloth for your altar, but it is not necessary. Using something you have (like a scarf or even a large cloth napkin) works as well.

3. Choose an item which will be in the center of your altar. This can be a candle, stone, statue, vase of flowers, inspirational photo, etc. Choose something that feels good to be the 'spoke of the wheel' of your altar. Imagine your altar like a radiating mandala, like a portal, like a cervix. What do you want in the center? What feels good? Try out several items. It's okay to switch items out if they do not end up feeling 'right'. Remember, there are no rules here!

4. Place other items surrounding the central item in whatever way flows out of you. I invite you not to think about it too hard. These are things which, when looked up and focused upon, bring you joy, inspiration, encouragement and happiness.

    a. You may also place items which represent that which you are releasing. These items will remind you of your intention to release said energies/qualities.

5. Once you have all of your items placed, sit back and gaze upon your altar. How does it feel when you gaze upon it? How does your body respond? How does your cervix respond? Notice the small voices of your body. If something doesn't feel 'right' about the way your altar is set up, change it.

6. Tend to your altar. As time goes on, your altar will get dirty, messed up, and will accumulate 'static' and 'gunk'. It is important to clean your altar at least every month. Wipe down

the items of dust. Wash the cloth. Change the water in the flowers. Remove and replace items which are no longer needed. An altar is a living thing. It is in constant transition, matching your own internal transition.

7. Enjoy the process!

SEVEN DAYS OF DAILY TOUCH

ONE of the primary ways to connect to your cervix is via touching your own cervix with your own hands. Most of the physical touch our cervix receives is from an Other (doctors and sexual partners). Women are taught that it is not okay for us to put our own fingers in ourselves, let alone touch our most innermost landscape.

For many Women, the cervix — the site of potential incredible pleasure — holds A LOT of pain. In order for the healing journey to reach its maximum potency, it is important for us to shine light on this pain. It is important to remember that which pains us, so as to release this stagnant energy from our cervix, and allow it to go back to the Earth.

The best way to do this is to dive into the ritual practice of touching your cervix with love and intention, and with your own fingers (and cut fingernails).

I invite you to do this in front of your altar and make it a sacred event. Light candles, play music you love, use essential oils or incense, get comfortable, and feel luxurious.

You do not need to touch your cervix for very long.

Explore what you notice, the longer you touch your cervix. What memories resurface? What triggers do you experience? What thoughts emerge? How does the rest of your body feel? Consciously witness yourself as you touch your cervix. All that arises is for healing. This is all part of the process.

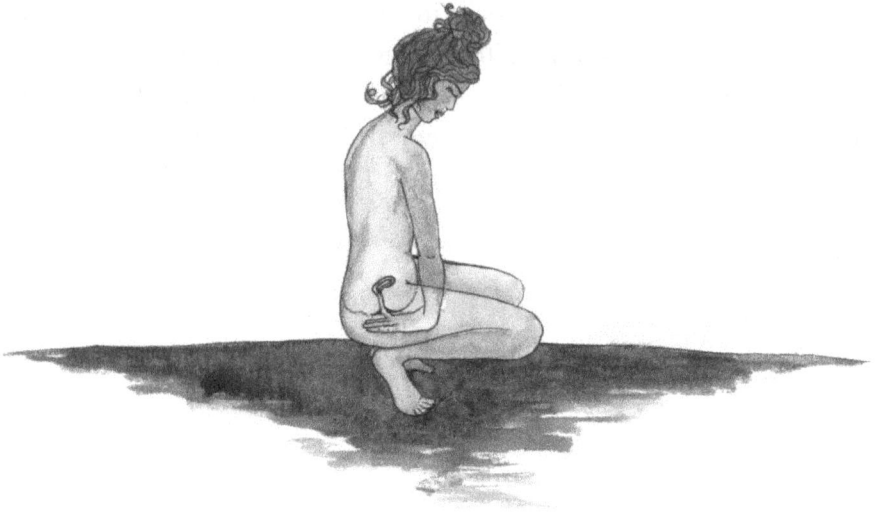

Sample 7-day Daily Touch Time Allotment + Focus

Day 1:   10 seconds
Focus on breathing
Day 2:   20 seconds
Focus on breathing and sensation
Day 3:   30 seconds
Focus on sensation and heart
Day 4:   30 seconds
Focus on heart and breathing
Day 5:   45 seconds
Focus on breathing, sensation and heart
Day 6:   1 min
Focus on breathing, sensation and heart
Day 7:   1 min
Focus on breathing

JOURNAL PROMPTS FOR
SELF-INQUIRY

U TILIZE these journal prompts throughout the duration of your

Cervical Wellness journey.

You may use the same prompts over and over again. Each time you do, more insights may be revealed.

What does the phrase 'sexual literacy' mean to me?

What do I know of my cervix?

When have I heard the voice of my cervix and didn't listen?

How can I begin to listen to the voice of my cervix?

What comes up when I touch my cervix?

What message is my cervix sending to me through abnormal paps?

What am I not wanting to see or feel?
What was my experience with sex ed?

What do I wish I had learned more about from sex ed?

How can I support myself to learn more?

When have I used my voice to stand up for my body?

What does the voice of my body sound/feel like?

What is my sexual history? What is my sexual timeline? (Write it all out)

(Looking at your timeline) What do I notice? How does this make me feel?

What is my gynecological history? What is my gynecological timeline? (Write it all out)

(Looking at your timeline) What do I notice? How does this make me feel?

What does self-advocacy mean to me?

What was the conversation like around sex in my family/ with my friends/ in my community?

How does my cervix want to be loved?

SAMPLE RECIPES FOR CERVICAL WELLNESS

Aᴌᴌ ingredients listed here are recommended to be of Organic, fair trade, and high-quality origin. We are what we eat, so why not choose to put the highest quality fuel into our bodies; especially, when we are healing or wanting to heal?

Remember, we want to BOOST OUR IMMUNE SYSTEM and the best way to do that is with food.

Flourless Breakfast Frittata

Preheat oven 350 degrees
Organic Ingredients
- 1 white onion
- 1 medium sized red bell pepper
- I cup spinach or kale
- ¼ cup basil
- Chicken-apple sausage (optional)
- 8-10 eggs (pastured and non-gmo preferred)
- ½ tsp Sea salt
- ½ tsp Fresh ground pepper

- Spices/herbs of your choice
- Coconut oil

- 12" cast iron pan

Finely chop onion and red bell pepper. Melt 1 tsp coconut oil in heated cast-iron pan, and sauté onion until it begins to turn translucent. Add bell pepper and continue to sauté. Cut sausage into small rounds or half/rounds and add to onion/pepper mix after 3 minutes. Finely chop spinach or kale (or any other green of your choice) and basil, and add to the pan.

While the greens are cooking down, crack and whisk together eggs, salt, pepper and herbs/spices of your choice into the egg mixture.

Pour egg mixture evenly into pan over sautéed vegetables and meat. Let cook over stove until the edges begin to firm up.

Once edges are firm, place the entire cast iron pan into the oven. Bake at 350 for 12-15 minutes, or until the egg is thoroughly cooked.

Serve immediately, or can be stored for reheating.

4-6 servings.

(Use this recipe as a template. Countless variations of vegetables, meats, spices and herbs can be used to create this flourless frittata to suit your exact taste!)

Butter Coffee/Tea
(Adapted from Bulletproof Coffee™)
Ingredients:
- Organic light roast coffee (tea may be substituted)
- 1 Tbsp Coconut oil (Nutiva is a good brand)
- 2 Tbsp Grass fed butter (Kerrygold Irish butter is good) or ghee
- ½ tsp Himalayan sea salt
- MCT Oil (optional)

- Cocoa powder (optional)
- Stevia (optional)

Blender/ Vitamix/ Hand Blender
Brew coffee using either drip or French press. Place all remaining ingredients into your blender/ vessel to blend. Pour coffee over. Blend until frothy. Drink while hot.
Serves 2-4
(This recipe is originally influenced by ghee tea as served in the high regions of Mongolia)

Collard Wraps

Ingredients:
- 1 bunch collard greens
- 1 avocado
- 1 tomato sliced
- Meat/meat substitute of choice
- Cheese (optional)
- ¼ red onion
- Cucumber — cut into spears
- Dressing of choice

Remove stalk/stem of 2-3 collard leaves. Place rest of ingredients in center of collard leave — layering like a burrito or sandwich. Roll up when complete. Can be wrapped in parchment paper/ reusable wax wrap paper and saved for later.
Serves 2-3
(Use this recipe as a template. Countless variations of vegetables, meats, spices and herbs can be used to create this collard wrap to suit your exact taste!)

Vegetable Soup Stock

Vegetable soup stock is one of the easiest things to make, and is super healthy for you, too! The trick is to save all your vegetable cuttings from cooking in a bag in a freezer. This includes onion skins, carrot peels, radish/beet/carrot tops, potato peels, celery ends, kale/chard stalks etc.

Once the bag is full or almost full, dump all contents into a soup pot. Fill with water. Bring to a boil. Lower temperature to bring to a simmer. Simmer for 1.5-2 hours.
Once complete, strain soup stock of vegetable matter with a colander. Now you have lots of vegetable stock to play with!

Bone Stock

Bone stock, whether made from beef/chicken/lamb/turkey bones, is one of the most nutritionally dense foods out there. High in minerals and saturated fat content (read Brain and Body food), bone broth is a necessary addition to any integrative healing regimen, and is super easy to make! The most difficult part is usually locating the bones. I invite and advise you to find a HIGH-QUALITY bone source — from grass fed/ pastured/ not tortured animals. You may pay a premium for them, but this being considered a medicine in my book, it is necessary to have only the top quality. The one trick to bone stock is the quality. Don't skimp on this.

Preheat oven to 425 degrees
Ingredients:
- Grass fed/pastured beef/chicken/lamb/turkey bones
- Carrots
- Onions
- Celery

- Ginger (optional)
- Turmeric (optional)
- Garlic (optional)
- 1-2 Bay leaves
- Any other immune-supporting herbs such as astragalus, turkey tail mushroom, osha root, etc.

Take bones out of packaging and place in a pot large enough to cover them with water. Cover with water, place on high heat and bring to a boil. Once brought to a boil, turn off heat and dump water out. This process 'cleans' the bones of any remaining blood or residue that you do not want in your stock. Do not skimp on this process. It is important for flavor and palatability.

Place bones on a baking sheet. Roughly cut up carrots, onions, celery, ginger, turmeric, and garlic (they do NOT need to be perfect, and can have the ends/skins on) and spread around bones on baking sheet. Place in oven and roast for 15-20 min or until bones begin to brown. Careful to not burn them. Check regularly.

Once done roasting, place all contents in a soup pot or crock pot. Pour boiling water into baking pan and with a wooden spoon, scrape off the browned remaining contents on the pan and pour into the pot. This adds a nice flavor to the stock. Cover bones and vegetables with water. Add bay leaves.

If in a crock pot, place on low and leave for a minimum of 24 hours. The longer, the better.

If in a soup pot, place on low, bring to a simmer, and leave for 8-10 hours. Again, the longer the better.

Once the time is up, strain contents out of broth. If you have beef or lamb bones, I invite you to scrape the marrow out of the bones and add it to the stock. This highly nutritional aspect of bones is a gold-mine for high quality fats, vitamins, and minerals.

Be aware that once the stock cools, there will be a thick lipid layer formed on the top. The liquid below may be gelatin –like from the collagen in the bones. When you go to use, be aware of this concentrate, and use with water to create the stock. Otherwise you can use the stock concentrate as it is, heat it up, and serve yourself a cup as medicine. Alternately, you can freeze the broth in ice cube trays to thaw out as needed.

Butternut Squash Soup

Preheat oven to 375 degrees

Ingredients:

- 1 med-large butternut squash
- 1 large onion
- 3-4 stalks celery
- 4 carrots
- 1 large yam
- 4 cups vegetable broth or bone broth or combination of both
- 2 tsp curry powder
- Salt and pepper to taste
- 2 Tbsp Coconut oil
- 1 can coconut milk
- Hand blender/ blender/ Vitamix

Put whole butternut squash on a baking pan and bake at 375 for 30 min or until tender to the touch. When you poke it, you should feel some give from the skin.

While waiting for the squash to cook, chop vegetables. In a large soup pot, combine onion and coconut oil. Sauté onion until it sweats. Add rest of vegetables and sauté in soup pot with coconut oil until they sweat.

When squash is tender to the touch, remove from oven and cut in half. Scoop out seeds and compost. Remove peel, cut into cubes and add to the vegetable mix in the soup pot. Stir together.

Add broth. Bring to a simmer, and cook until yams and carrots are tender and soft.

Remove from heat. Add coconut milk, salt, pepper and curry powder. With a hand blender or in a blender, puree the chunky soup until smooth, or until consistency you prefer. Sometimes it is nice to leave chunks of vegetables, or you can blend it until homogenous and smooth.

Garnish with parmesan cheese, Greek yogurt, sour cream or have as is.

SAMPLE RECIPES FOR CERVICAL WELLNESS

Over the past three years I have worked 1:1 with countless Women on their Cervical Wellness Healing Journeys. Throughout our time together, many of the Women I work with bring to my attention alternate resources, recipes, and ideas of which I was not aware beforehand. It is my pleasure to share with you other helpful resources that have been shared with me. I truly believe the more information and options we have for our reproductive health, the better.

Without further ado, here are MORE goodies to support you in your Cervical Wellness Healing Journey.

Coconut Oil + Essential Oil Suppository

- Combine 3 Tbsp coconut oil, 20 drops lemon essential oil, 40 drops lemongrass essential oil
- Melt and blend all together
- Pour into small ice cube trays and freeze to harden
- Place one inside of your vaginal canal as close to the cervix as you can get right before bed

- Do this while sleeping to prevent the oil from leaking out. As well, I recommend wearing a panty-liner to protect your underwear
- *My client reported that this made a great lubricant as well — Fun and healing all wrapped into one!*

Herbal Regimen as Advised by a Naturopathic Doctor

Ingredients:

Echinacea angustifolia root (NEVER purpurea)
Vegetable glycerine
Usnea Tincture
Calendula Tincture

Protocol:

Powder the root as finely as flour (use a nut or coffee grinder for the last stages) Blend it with vegetable glycerine until it is the consistency of bread dough; you may need to add flour to keep it from being sticky. Make 14 lozenges about the size of your thumb. Place them on a tray and put in the freezer (they will be too soft otherwise). Once frozen, take one and place it against the cervix every night for 14 nights.

The next morning, douche with a combination of usnea tincture, calendula tincture, and water (about 1 tsp of each of the tinctures). This protocol will be greatly aided by some guided imagery meditation which helps you to visualize the healing.

CHAPTER ELEVEN
FURTHER RESOURCES

IF you are interested in seeing if there is a wild source of water near you, head to www.findaspring.com. They have an interactive map of the USA showing all the places where you can harvest your own natural spring water.

You can purchase loose, raw herbs at your local apothecary or online at www.mountainroseherbs.com. For tincture and oil, I recommend going to www.herb-pharm.com.

Cervical Self-Exam Kits: http://beautifulcervix.com/see-your-own-beautiful-cervix/

Crystals for intra-vaginal use: www.yonicrystals.love

Fertility Awareness Method: www.tcoyf.com

Learn more about dearmoring the cervix and awakening cervical pleasure at: https://selfcervix.com/

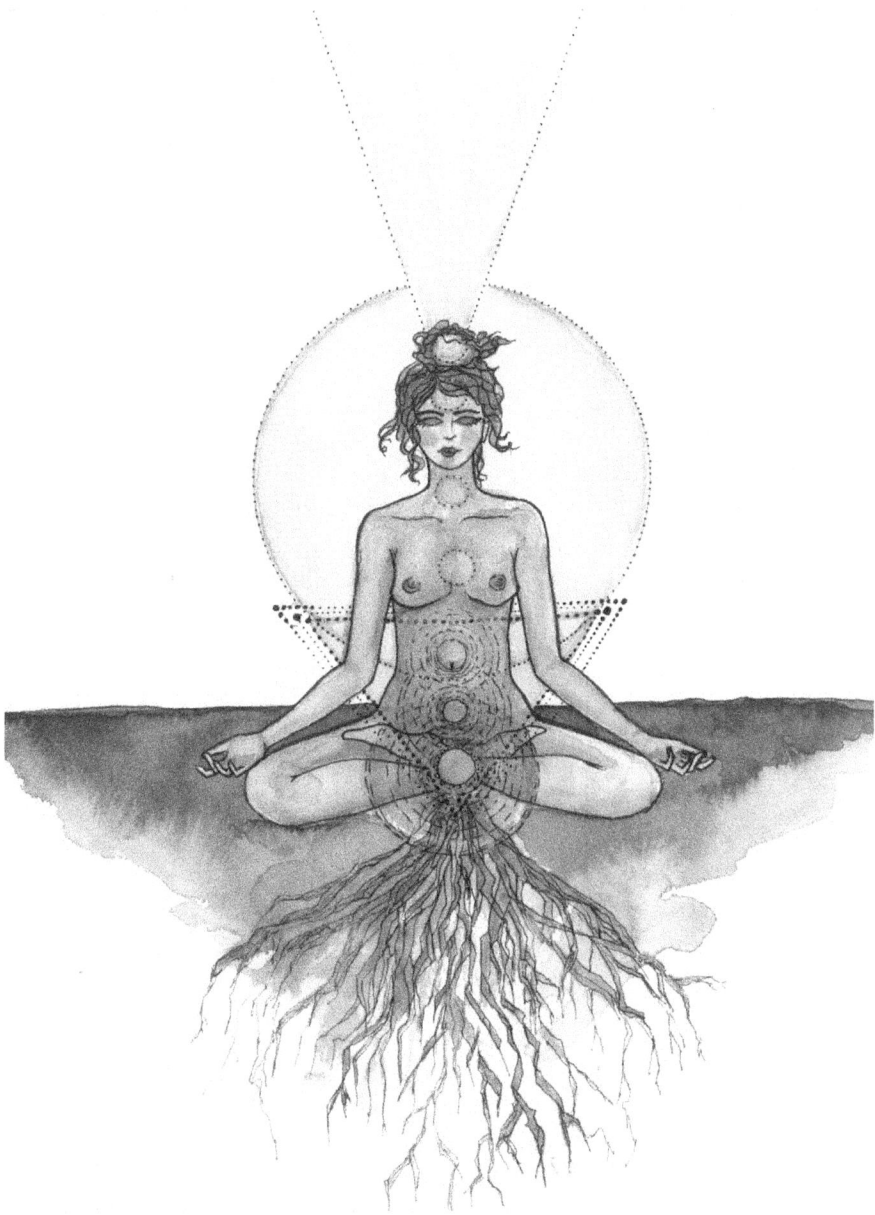

CONCLUSION

LAST night was Halloween/ Samhain/ All Hallows Eve and instead of doing the usual 'dress up in a costume and go to a party', I decided to tap into the sacred. I made a fire in my outdoor fire pit and laid a blanket down alongside it. I held in my hand the mushrooms I was to ingest and called upon my Grandmothers to be there with me as I communed with the plant medicine. I ate the mushrooms just as the sun dipped below the horizon and set off on an inward journey. I know this book is about neither mushroom medicine nor Halloween, but the experience I had over the course of the next five hours solidified my knowing that this work — the work of healing our connection to our bodies and our cervix — is imperative for the healing of our planet.

On this journey I was met by Spider Woman, the great weaver and creatrix of the Universe and Life. In mythos around the world,

Spider Woman is considered the great Goddess; the great Mother whose web connects all living Beings to one another. It is said she emerged out of the great void and within her body and through the weaving of her web, all of the bodies of this Universe were born. She is, in essence, the one who created us all.

Spider Woman showed me how the untimely deaths from disease (like cancer) of the Women of this world stem not from anything that's been done in their lives, but rather, what *hasn't* been done. I saw how, within the female body, lies the foundation of creation; the smoldering fire through which new life is manifested. This Dark Feminine essence inside us all has been repressed and suppressed to such a degree that this energy has become corrosive and putrid. It's had no room for expression in this world for the past two millennia and because of this, has begun to turn on us.

Time and time again I get asked the question, 'Why doesn't HPV affect men the same way it affects women?" I now have an answer to this.

Contraction of the HPV virus and the development of cervical dysplasia which follows is a reminder to us that we've forgotten our dark feminine essence. Our immune system is the final hope of our body to remain unscathed from this forgetting and repression, and when that goes down through lack of boundaries/ poor lifestyle choices/ chronic stress, we're left defenseless. The cervix, the anchor to our dark-feminine, is the bridge between our inner and outer worlds, and the forgetting of this truth is what causes damage and produces abnormalities. The energy of our dark feminine essence is looking for a place to express, but is turned to poison and seeps out through our cervix.

Male bodies hold the dark feminine within them because they're born from a female body, but not to the degree that females do. Our uterus, our womb, is the smoldering cauldron of creation and our cervix is the portal through which these creations are born.

Can you see how this forgetting; this repression on the part of our society, our religions and our cultural structure has cultivated an atmosphere where the female body turns against itself? The portrayal of the dark being 'evil', 'bad', and 'scary' has caused generations of women to reject their bodies and who *they really are* — the keepers of the sacred portal of Life and Death. From the darkness Life is created and back to the darkness we return upon Death. This not scary. It is sacred. And true.

Things are changing, and every Woman in my life can feel it too.

We as Women in this time are creating and birthing a new world. This creation and birthing stems from the fires of transmutation, and Cervical Wellness is but a single node of the great web we're weaving with this new era. Cervical Wellness within the pathway of self-healing stands as an anchor-point through which we can transform.

Whether you've read this book because you have HPV and cervical dysplasia, are a women's health and wellness practitioner, know someone in your life who is dealing with these conditions, or for any other reason, know that this work will change you. It will change you when you realize how much you weren't told. It will change you when you realize how much was kept from us as we were growing into adulthood. It will also change you when you come to remember and take action.

This book *is* the fire of transmutation.

You've made it this far. You now *know* the truth of the magic of your body. You *know* that you can heal yourself, because you have the vital life force of our world running through you. And now that you know, I call upon you to spread the word.

Help me weave a new web, like the great Spider Woman, where the female body is honored and revered for the role it plays in our world. Help me embody the voice of the cervix; the sacred portal inside us all.

Help me by helping and healing yourself, against all the odds every Western medical doctor has placed on you. Do not believe them. They're not the authority over your body: You are, and you alone.

This is a call out to all my Sisters to stand up and say, 'No more, no more this way.' Together we are weaving a new world; a Women's Web of Change where at the web's center resides the cervix, growing and regenerating in all her sacred glory.

Together, we are healing our bodies. Together, we are healing the Earth. When we heal, the world around us heals. This is how we initiate the change so many of us long for.

This is the work of our time. This is the work of our lifetime.

We've got this. And I'll be here, continuously believing in you.

I believe in us all.

Let's do this.

REFERENCES | ENDNOTES

Behbakht, K., Friedman, J., Heimler, I., Aroutcheva, A., Simoes, J., & Faro, S. (2014). Role of the Vaginal Microbiological Ecosystem and Cytokine Profile in the Promotion of Cervical Dysplasia: A Case–Control Study. *Infectious Diseases in Obstetrics & Gynecology*, (10), 181-186.

Beverly Whipple & Barry R. Komisaruk (2002) Brain (PET) Responses to Vaginal-Cervical Self-Stimulation in Women with Complete Spinal Cord Injury: Preliminary Findings, Journal of Sex & Marital Therapy, 28:1, 79-86, DOI: 10.1080/009262302317251043

Chavalier, G. (2007). The Earth's electrical surface potential A summary of present understanding. Retrieved from http://www.protyposis.info/dokumente/earthwaver/earthwaver-studie--chevalier--source-of-earthspotential.pdf

Chung, S., Franceschi, S., & Lambert, P. (2008). Estrogen and ERα: Culprits in cervical cancer? *Trends in Endocrinology & Metabolism,* 504-511.

Fang, C., Miller, S., Bovbjerg, D., Bergman, C., Edelson, M., Rosenblum, N., . . . Douglas, S. (2008). Perceived Stress is Associated with Impaired T-Cell Response to HPV16 in Women with Cervical Dysplasia. *Annals of Behavioral Medicine,* 87-96

Li, Q., & Kawada, T. (2009). *Healthy forest parks make healthy people: Forest environments enhance human immune function.* Department of Hygiene and Health, Tokyo: Nippon Medical School. Retrieved April 20, 2015, from http://www.hphpcentral.com/wp-content/uploads/2010/09/5000-paper-by-Qing-Li2-2.pdf

Scheurer, M., Danysh, H., Follen, M., & Lupon, P. (2014). Association of traffic-related hazardous air pollutants and cervical dysplasia in an urban multiethnic population: A cross-sectional study. *Environmental Health, 13*(52). Retrieved April 21, 2015, from http://www.ehjournal.net/content/13/1/52

What is HPV? (2015, January 22). Retrieved April 29, 2015, from http://www.cdc.gov/hpv/whatishpv.html

Yardley, K. (2001). Understanding Cervical Dysplasia: A Holistic Treatment Protocol. *British Journal of Phytotherapy, 5*(4)

---

[1] Dr. George Nicholaus Papanicolaou, http://papsociety.org/gpbio.html, 6/25/18

[2] HPV Vaccine, http://www.hpvvaccine.org.au/parents/how-long-does-it-take-for-hpv-cancers-to-develop.aspx

[3] What is HPV? (2015, January 22). Retrieved April 29, 2015, from http://www.cdc.gov/hpv/whatishpv.html

[4] Ibid

[5] Ibid

[6] Yardley, K. (2001). Understanding Cervical Dysplasia: A Holistic Treatment Protocol. *British Journal of Phytotherapy*, 5(4)

[7] Ibid

[8] University of Copenhagen. "How Viruses Make Body Cells Work For Them." ScienceDaily. ScienceDaily, 2 April 2007. <www.sciencedaily.com/releases/2007/03/070330100654.htm>.

[9] Ibid

[10] Prochaska, J.O., DiClemente, C.C., & Norcross, J.C. (1992). In search of how people change: Applications to the addictive behaviors. American Psychologist, 47, 1102-1114. PMID: 1329589.

[11] https://www.prochange.com/transtheoretical-model-of-behavior-change

[12] Mills, S. (1993). *The essential book of herbal medicine*. London: Arkana.

[13] Micozzi, M. (2014). Western Herbalism. In *Fundamentals of Complementary and Alternative Medicine* (5th ed.). London: Elsevier Health Sciences.

[14] Del Priore G[1], Gudipudi DK, Montemarano N, Restivo AM, Malanowska-Stega J, Arslan AA., Oral diindolylmethane (DIM): pilot evaluation of a nonsurgical treatment for cervical dysplasia. Gynecol Oncol. 2010 Mar;116(3):464-7. doi: 10.1016/j.ygyno.2009.10.060. Epub 2009 Nov 24.

[15] Fang, C., Miller, S., Bovbjerg, D., Bergman, C., Edelson, M., Rosenblum, N., . . . Douglas, S. (2008). Perceived Stress is Associated

with Impaired T-Cell Response to HPV16 in Women with Cervical Dysplasia. *Annals of Behavioral Medicine*, 87-96

[16] https://www.cdc.gov/cancer/cervical/basic_info/risk_factors.htm

[17] ibid

[18] Chung, S., Franceschi, S., & Lambert, P. (2008). Estrogen and ERα: Culprits in cervical cancer? Trends in Endocrinology & Metabolism, 504-511.

[19] Li, Q., & Kawada, T. (2009). Healthy forest parks make healthy people: Forest environments enhance human immune function. Department of Hygiene and Health, Tokyo: Nippon Medical School. Retrieved April 20, 2015, from http://www.hphpcentral.com/wp-content/uploads/2010/09/5000-paper-by-Qing-Li2-2.pdf

[20] Babak A. Ardekani, Khadija Figarsky, John J. Sidtis; Sexual Dimorphism in the Human Corpus Callosum: An MRI Study Using the OASIS Brain Database, *Cerebral Cortex*, Volume 23, Issue 10, 1 October 2013, Pages 2514–2520, https://doi.org/10.1093/cercor/bhs253

[21] Allen, Richey, Chai, Gorski; Sex Differences in the Corpus Callosum of the Living Human Being, *The Journal of Neuroscience*, 11(4), April 1991: 933-942

[22] Sigurdardotti, Elisabet; Women and Madness in the 19th Century — The effects of oppression on women's mental health; Sept 2013, Hasholi Islands

[23] (https://www.cbsnews.com/news/metoo-reaches-85-countries-with-1-7-million-tweets/)

[24] (https://www.cbsnews.com/news/metoo-more-than-12-million-facebook-posts-comments-reactions-24-hours/).

[25] https://en.wikipedia.org/wiki/Colposcopy 6/1/18

[26] Halioua, Bruno MD, "The Participation of Hans Hinselmann in Medical Experiments at Auschwitz", Journal of Lower Genital Tract

Disease: January 2010 - Volume 14 - Issue 1 - p 1-4 doi:
10.1097/LGT.0b013e3181af30ef

GLOSSARY

Adaptive immune system: The part of the immune system found at the cellular level which produces antibodies to kill off pathogens and stop their growth. Also known as the 'acquired immune system'.

Allopathic medicine: A style of medicine that uses treatments and remedies to cure diseases. The style of medicine practiced in most Western hospitals and clinics.

Altruism: Putting the care and concern of others as a top priority.

Behavior: Actions and mannerisms of an individual.

Bioelectricity: The electrical currents found in living organisms and systems.

Blacks Lives Matter: An international activist movement which campaigns against violence and systematic racism towards black people.

Carcinoma in-situ: A group of abnormal cells described as a cancer that is only present in the cells where it originated and has not spread. There exists some disagreement around whether or not to describe this as 'cancer'.

Cis-hetero (Cis-heterosexual): A heterosexual person who personally identifies with the gender they were assigned at birth.

Colposcopy: A procedure using a colposcope to get a closer look at the cervix, usually performed after an abnormal pap-test result. Biopsies of the cervix are taken for analysis.

Dysplasia: Abnormal cell growth.

Eclampsia: A life-threatening condition of seizures caused by high-blood pressure following giving birth.

Effacement: The process of the cervix to prepare for delivery of a baby. The cervix thins as dilation occurs and the baby's head descends towards the birth canal.

Gynecology: In medicine it refers to the practice dealing with the health of the female reproductive system (vagina, uterus, ovaries) and breasts. Outside medicine it means 'the science of women'.

Innate immune system: The part of the immune system that is made up of barriers meant to keep bacteria, viruses, parasites, etc. outside of the body.

Pap-smear: An exam used to test for precancer and cancer on the cervix.

Parasympathetic nervous response: 'Rest and digest' function of the nervous system.

Perseverance: A steady and consistent course of action towards a goal or purpose in spite of obstacles, follies or hardships.

Plant spirit medicine: A way of working with plants that recognizes and honors the higher-intelligence and non-physical benefits of the individual plant.

Regenerate: The process of renewal, growth and restoration.

Self-healing: The process of recovery that is motivated and directed by the instinct of the patient themselves.

Sympathetic nervous response: 'Fight, flight, freeze" function of the nervous system.

Western medicine: The treatment of medical conditions by doctors with medications and treatments according to Western scientific standards.

List of Abbreviations

CIN: Cervical Intraepithelial Neoplasia, also known as cervical dysplasia

LEEP: Loop Electrosurgical Excision Procedure

STI: Sexually Transmitted Infection

INDEX

ACKNOWLEDGMENTS

A book like this warrants many acknowledgments. I see them all as Angels who've beckoned me to use my voice and share my truth with all the courage I could muster. The subject matter is raw and vulnerable, and there has been no end of individuals along the way who've supported and championed me to continue on and share this with the world, even though every fiber of my Being has wanted to run away from it all several times.

Thank you to my publisher Smokeblood Publishing for believing in this work and helping me spread the voice of the cervix far and wide.

Thank you to Hillary Mendoza for your incredible artistic contribution to this book.

Thank you, Dr. Susie Dehnad, OBGYN of Sutter Medical in Santa Rosa, CA. That fateful day you told me there was nothing else the medical system could do for me was one of the most difficult, yet catalyzing, days of my life. Thank you for unknowingly thrusting me into my healing journey.

Thank you, Dr. Christiane Northrup, MD for writing the book *Women's Body, Women's Wisdom,* from which fell the beginning breadcrumbs that guided me towards the journey of healing myself. Your book has been my number one, go-to resource for empowering Women's Health-based information.

Thank you to Phyllis Bala, Doctor of Indigenous Medicine: A Medical intuitive, and one of the most profound teachers I've ever had. You opened the doorway for me to fully dive into the magic and medicine found within my inner world. Thank you for being a pivotal turning point in my healing journey.

Thank you to Dr. Mirie Levy, professor of Health Education from my final semester at the California Institute of Integral Studies. It was your assignments that gave me the opportunity to coalesce all that I'd learned while healing my cervix, and share it with a group of Women. I received my first clear pap-result of seven years during that semester, and through your course, was able to celebrate that achievement.

Thank you to my entire CIIS graduating cohort, MA in Integrative Health Studies, class of 2016. Together we survived the rigor of grad school, through which I cultivated the discipline to complete this book. Also, much of what I learned about health, healing and wellness happened alongside all of you, making each and every one of you very much a part of the story, too.

Thank you to Marissa Waraksa, editor and guide through the molding of this manuscript. Thank you for your courage in asking for the trade of taking part in my Sacred Portal online program, in exchange for editing this creation. I am forever grateful for your keen eye and direct communication style. It truly helped me to make it to the finish line.

Thank you to each and every one of my incredible lady friends, who've supported me all along this way, and throughout the years. There were so many times when I felt scared to speak about this project, feeling I would be 'too much', but you listened and reflected back to me only enthusiasm and encouragement. Thank you Sena Shellenberger, Meredith Rom, Karen Prosen, Anne-Louise Cole, Stirling Freeman, and many, many others.

Thank you to Nick and Teresa Randall, my soon-to-be in-laws and landlords. What a gift it's been to live on your land in a house worth much more than we pay. The beauty surrounding me at all times in this home has provided me the mental space and fresh air to feel resourced enough to take on this project. This home has held me the whole time. I'm so, so grateful.

Thank you to my cat-family — Apollo, Artemis, Sammy, and Flower — for enduring my endless outpouring of affection onto you, and providing consistent entertainment and love. I appreciate how often you've sat on or beside me as I worked on this manuscript.

Thank you to my amazing family: my Mother Loretta, father Gregg and sister Debra, for always believing in me and accepting me for who I am. Thank you for standing by me, even when I was unstable and afraid. Thank you for always having my back and for loving me so deeply. I love you too.

Thank you to my Beloved John-Nicholas Randall, my other whole and teammate for life. Your devotion to me and to our relationship provided me with a safe container for the healing journey of my cervix. You were there throughout my entire process of healing. All these years, you changed alongside me, and adopted the lifestyle necessary for me to heal. I really don't know if I could've done *any* of this without you — healing, grad-school, writing this book, Cervical Wellness as a whole, entrepreneurship — all of these accomplishments occurred because I had your unwavering support. You're a rock in my sea of immense feeling. Words can never express how deeply I love you.

Finally, I absolutely must thank Alakshia, the true voice of the book. Call Alakshia an Angel, a higher-dimensional Being, an imaginary friend, a voice in my head, a spirit guide, energy, or whatever else you call a non-tangible intelligence that is outside our general spectrum of perception, but there was definitely an Other who guided me in this process. I can't tell you how many times I tried to stop, attempting to cease the continuous flood of information and inspiration because I wanted to do something else. I didn't *want* to talk about the cervix and Women's health all the time. I *wanted* to talk about the forest, and medicine from nature. Every time I'd throw in the towel, however; Alakshia poked and prodded me from the inside, to continue on. On a few occasions, I became physically unwell with strange symptoms, and they'd subside and go away only when I'd pick Cervical Wellness back on up, and continue on. Only when I fully surrendered and acquiesced to this energy, did the flow lead me to the completion of this book. I had to give in, and let Alakshia in.

Right now, as I'm typing this, I'm realizing that maybe Alakshia isn't some outside energy propelling me forward, but that Alakshia is actually my Body, and that the voice I've been hearing and listening to is that of my very own Body.

Thank you, Body. Thank you for being my vehicle in this life, and for proving to me that magic is real. Thank you for remembering with me that we Humans are far more powerful and capable than we've been led to believe.

Thank you, Ancestors, thank you GrandMothers. Thank you Ayahuasca, for opening me up to the collective grief and pain of my GrandMothers; for all the pain and trauma of their cervix that was left unexpressed upon their death. This book is in their honor. May Women no longer be left in the dark in regard to the beauty and sanctity of their own bodies.

Thank you, Earth, and all the other members of the Web of Life. I do this for you, in your honor. May we remember our own place in this sacred web. May we all heal, and bring balance once more to this incredible planet.

Thank you, Sun, for your life-giving energy. Thank you for your light and warmth. Thank you for animating me.

Thank you, Moon, for always lighting up the dark, or hiding so I could see my own shadows.

Thank you, Water, for your Life (and all the gourds of Máte you filled, which fueled the endless hours on my computer).

Thank you, Great Spirit, that which is greater than Me.
Thank you, Universe.
Thank you, Life.

ABOUT THE AUTHOR

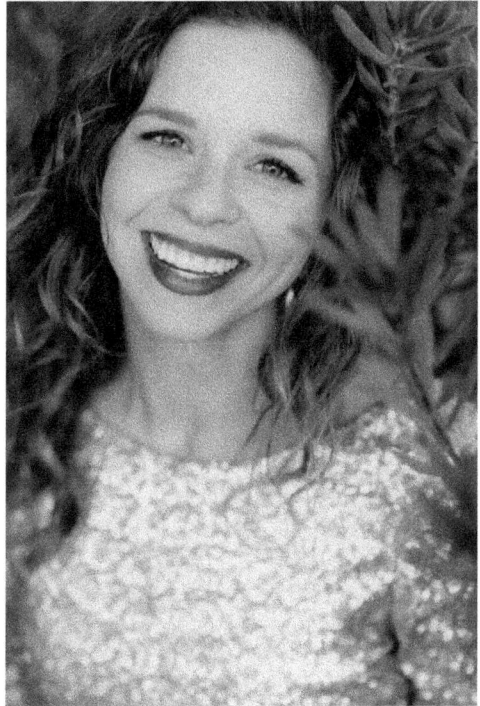

Denell Nawrocki, MA is a guide, speaker, and teacher specializing in Women's wellness and Earth-based health. She believes in the body's ability to heal, and guides Women to connect to their body to find empowerment on the self-healing path.

Since 2008, Denell has done extensive study in the fields of holistic health, healing, personal transformation, indigenous wisdom, plant medicine and history. All of this culminates in her mission to lead people to be in loving relationship with their body and Earth in order to repair the Sacred Web of Life. She received her MA in Integrative Health Studies from California Institute of Integral Studies (CIIS), and a BA in History from UC Davis.

Utilizing all she studied, Denell self-healed 7 years of HPV and cervical dysplasia and has retained a clear bill of health ever since. In 2016, Denell founded Cervical Wellness, an online-education platform guiding Women to self-heal from HPV and cervical dysplasia, as well as reconnect to their female sacred-anatomy in new and empowering ways.

She offers online courses & events, in-person workshops & retreats, as well as sharing illuminating content in public talks, and on Instagram & YouTube. Find her and her work at www.cervicalwellness.com

ABOUT THE PUBLISHER

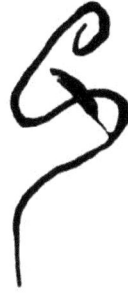

Smokeblood Publishing is a mythopoetic collective that strives to seek out, absorb and disseminate creative excellence in the written word.

"The whole thing is a weaving of smoke." -Alan Watts

If you'd like to publish your own book, or for bulk discounts, please contact the publisher directly:

IG: @_smokeblood

Email: connect@smokebloodpublishing.com

Website: www.smokeblood.com

www.ingramcontent.com/pod-product-compliance
Lightning Source LLC
Chambersburg PA
CBHW072118020426
42334CB00018B/1641